What readers are saying about *Doing Well at Being Sick...*

You've heard that we learn more in the valleys than on the mountaintops. Wendy Wallace has lived this maxim... *Doing Well at Being Sick* tugs at your heart, yet tickles your funny bone. You're about to... draw wisdom, perspective, and hope from a great, gifted, and godly woman. — **John D. Beckett, Chairman, The Beckett Companies, Author of** *Loving Monday* **and** *Mastering Monday*

In my several decades of practice in Internal Medicine and Cardiology I have seen no one with as long a list of diverse and often unrelated major medical problems remain so full of life and appreciation for every day. Wendy has created a wonderful reading experience for patients, support persons, and health providers... and I am sure that the patient community around the country is going to find it extremely valuable. — **Melvyn Rubenfire, MD, Professor of Internal Medicine, Director of Preventive Cardiology, University of Michigan**

Wendy's faith, wisdom, and friendship have not only inspired me as a nurse... but have directly influenced my life, family, future, and spiritual and ministerial growth... *Doing Well at Being Sick* introduces the reader to a magnificent woman, and illustrates her journey through incredible health crises and personal challenges, utilizing common sense, personal responsibility, biblical scholarship, and divine grace as guidance. — **Pamela F. Stevenson RN, BSN, MPS, Practice Management Coordinator, University of Michigan Medical Center**

This book is the rare combination of practical tools, biblical wisdom, and sweet companionship for those who walk the lonely road of chronic illness, as well as for those who love and support them. — **Shelly Beach, author of** *Precious Lord, Take My Hand* **and** *Ambushed by Grace*

This is a wonderful, inspirational work that should help any patient maneuvering the health-care system succeed in overcoming the many challenges of having a chronic illness. — **W. Joseph McCune, MD, Michael H. and Marcia S. Klein Professor of Rheumatic Diseases, University of Michigan**

Wendy's book is not about surviving illness. It is about the emotional, physical, and spiritual growth of a triumphant life that has been filled with hope, healing, and inspiration. Her writing takes us inside her journey and at the same time offers practical advice for anyone suffering illness and for those who love them. It is rare to find a book that teaches and touches the reader. This is such a book. — **Robert J. Ackerman, PhD, Professor and Director of the Mid-Atlantic Addiction Research & Training Institute at Indiana University of Pennsylvania, and a co-founder of the National Association for Children of Alcoholics**

Wendy Wallace's personal experience in living well with long-term illness provides wisdom for the healthy and the sick. This book should be a benefit covered by health insurance. — **Tanya Strong, RN, BSN, wife and mother of three, doing well with mixed-connective tissue disease**

Inspirational and informative to others with chronic disease. The information on how to negotiate the health-care system, dealing with physicians, and all the frustrations encountered are on target. What I appreciate most is that Wendy gives people solutions to these challenges. — **Carole Dodge, OTR, CHT, University of Michigan Department of Physical Medicine and Rehabilitation**

Doing Well at Being Sick is chock-full of practical and useful ideas... The amalgam of her personal health journey, useful tools for navigating the health system, and the overriding spiritual aspects is potent and powerful. — **Sherri Plank, educator, who also cared for her mother through decades of multiple physical challenges**

As someone who works in the world of medical care, I am impressed by the reality described by Wendy Wallace. Sometimes that medical reality is chilling, sometimes it is heartwarming, but it is always worth our attention. I recommend this book to both medical professionals and patients. — **Spencer Maidlow, President/CEO of Covenant HealthCare System, Saginaw, Michigan; current President of Michigan Hospital Association**

DOING WELL
at BEING SICK

Living with Chronic and Acute Illness

Wendy Wallace

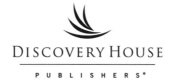

DISCOVERY HOUSE
PUBLISHERS®

Discovery House books are distributed to the trade exclusively by
Barbour Publishing, Inc., Uhrichsville, Ohio.

Requests for permission to quote from this book should be directed
to: Permissions Department, Discovery House Publishers, P.O. Box
3566, Grand Rapids, MI 49501.

Interior design by Sherri L. Hoffman

Library of Congress Cataloging-in-Publication Data
Wallace, Wendy Drew
    Doing well at being sick : living with chronic and acute
illness / Wendy Wallace.
        p.   cm.
Includes bibliographical references and index.
ISBN 978-1-57293-387-3 (alk. paper)
    1. Sick—Psychology. 2. Chronic diseases—Religious
aspects. I. Title.
R726.5.W353 2010
616'.044—dc22   2010020608

Printed in the United States of America

10 11 12 13 14 / 10 9 8 7 6 5 4 3 2 1

I thank God for showering me with His grace and love,
especially through Rick, Carey, and Mark,
the three most remarkable people I have ever known.
We have lived this together.

Contents

~

Acknowledgments

*"Praise the Lord, O my soul, and forget
not all his benefits" (Psalm 103:2).*

I would never have been able to do well at being sick without the loving support and encouragement of many friends and family members, especially our Bible study and church family. To list you all would be to double the length of the book and risk my editor's wrath. I have tried to thank you along our way together. God has certainly blessed us with your love.

My special editors, Rick, Carey, and Mark Wallace, read and commented on the book line by line. They are all gifted writers in their own rights, and their painstaking advice was invaluable. When I was tired, they prayed for me; when I did not want to keep writing, they encouraged me; when I was sick, they cared for me; when I was unclear about how to express something, they talked it through with me. *Doing Well* would not exist without them.

I also want to thank the other people who read the manuscript and offered me wonderful focused comments, often spending hours in this process. Many of them have been friends for decades, and I truly appreciate the care they spent making *Doing Well* a better tool for readers. Thank you to:

Robert Ackerman, Shelly Beach, Fred Bean, John Beckett, Debbie Boyce, Wendy Cole, Carol Dodge, George Gallup, Ethel Jensen, James Leonard, Spencer Maidlow, W. Joseph McCune, Chris Newhouse, Sheryl Plank, Melvyn Rubenfire, Felix Scheffel,

Quentin Schultze, Nancy Schumann, Pamela Stevenson, Tanya Strong, Diane Telian, and Catherine Varner.

The Discovery House staff has added their considerable talents to bringing the project to fruition, including Judith Markham, Annette Gysen, and Katy Pent. I am especially grateful that Quentin Schultze introduced me to Carol Holquist, whose encouragement and advice guided the writing even before we had a formal contract. Carol's walk with God through the challenges of this life inspires me to continue to do well.

We thank God for all of you.

Preface

*Y*ou are probably reading this because you or someone you love struggles with a serious health problem. I know how you feel, and I want to help. *Doing Well at Being Sick* tells the story of my life with both chronic and acute illness for over twenty years. But I don't concentrate on aches and pains. Instead, I share practical information I've learned about how to live a full life despite the hard realities of illness.

At age forty-seven and in relatively good health, I had a lupus-related heart attack that damaged one-third of my heart muscle. As my family and I struggled to recover from that shock, I had a second heart attack one week later. In the next eighteen months I faced lung cancer, chemotherapy, gall bladder disease, colon cancer, three surgeries, and another heart attack. Our family joked that we funded a new wing in the hospital that year. Since then I have had three more heart attacks, bladder cancer, major skin cancer, trigeminal neuralgia, and many more diagnoses and surgeries, all while coping with the exhaustion and constant pain associated with lupus and degenerative arthritis. I have learned not only to manage my illness but also to draw my strength from God and live a joyful life.

My experience enables me to answer questions often asked by patients and families who face chronic illness:

- Where can you find strength on days when all you experience is weakness?
- What do you do with the guilt that comes from burdening those you love?

- How can you trust God when things seem to be going wrong?
- How do you handle your inability to do what you used to do?
- How can you help your friends and family to cope with your illness?
- What can you do to assist your doctors in giving you the best care?
- How do you forgive medical professionals when they make serious mistakes?

None of us would choose to live with illness. But the sickness brings us opportunities. We can use the pain to learn about what is important in life. We can practice praising instead of complaining. We can explore what will bring lasting peace to us and our loved ones as well as glory to God.

Why am I still alive and functioning? God's grace, the love and support of friends and family, and hard-earned knowledge in navigating the medical system have taught me to do well at being sick. I hope to help you do the same.

Chapter One

Admitting You Are Sick:
What Happens Next?

You will learn:

- to ask questions until you have answers that will help you face challenges
- to apply God's grace to your medical care
- to accept God's sovereignty over your health
- to embrace new tasks for your new self
- to believe that you can do well at living with sickness

Through many dangers, toils and snares
I have already come;
'Tis grace hath brought me safe thus far,
And grace will lead me home.

~JOHN NEWTON

The green lines varied little as they ran across the television screen, but they fascinated me. This was my heart beating, something I had taken for granted until a few hours earlier.

I ignored the chest pains when they started the day before. I had spent the week in a small town outside of St. Louis running a training group for executives of a large corporation. I thought I was having a bad reaction to a new allergy medicine and asked my training partner, Ralph, to take over our group while I took some antacids. The antacids didn't work, and the pain got worse. Just after midnight Ralph put me in the rental car and took me to the emergency room of the local hospital.

I have always had a high pain tolerance. Once, when I was a little girl, my mother stuck a thermometer in my mouth to keep me quiet while she nursed my sister's flu and discovered that my fever was four degrees higher than my sister's. The ER doctor asked me a standard set of questions, and by the time he finished I felt like the proverbial elephant was sitting on my chest. I tried to remain calm to help the doctor in diagnosing my pain, but when he asked me to rate it from 1 to 10, I said 10, the worst I had ever experienced, including childbirth.

The doctor didn't believe me. He told me that I had indigestion and should go home and get a good night's sleep. I started to cry, feeling hopeless to explain to this man what the situation really was inside my body. Ralph took the doctor aside. "I know this woman very well. If she says she is in pain, she's in pain," he told the doctor. "You *will* admit her." Ralph's calm insistence coupled with his 6'6" presence saved my life.

The doctor reluctantly agreed that he had much to lose if he was wrong and little to lose if Ralph was wrong. The only bed available at the time was in the intensive care unit. The moment the nurses hooked me up to the monitors, the ICU staff jumped into action; I was having a major heart attack.

By the time my enzyme levels came back from the laboratory several hours later, thirty percent of my heart had essentially died.

Early that morning I called my family in Michigan. My fifteen-year-old son, Mark, answered the phone, and I asked for my husband, Rick. Mark said Dad had left for work early that morning, so I had Mark wake our daughter, Carey. It was Carey's eighteenth birthday, and I was supposed to be flying home in a few hours to celebrate. Instead we were having a conversation I never dreamed we would have.

Carey sounded sleepy and a little grumpy. "Are you still going to be home in time for my birthday dinner tonight?"

"Actually, that is why I am calling. I am in the hospital having a heart attack, but I am okay. I love you all." We cried and talked for a few minutes until I said, "I think I'd better call Dad now." When I reached him at the office, Rick excitedly started to tell me about a great development at his work, but I interrupted to tell him about the heart attack. He called the kids, told Carey to pack some things for him, and caught the first plane to St. Louis, alternately praying and crying the entire way. When he arrived at my bedside, I burst into tears, told him I loved him, and made him promise me to take good care of the kids if I didn't live. He, of course, promised, but I wasn't satisfied. "Really listen to them. Don't sort the mail while they are talking to you." Funny the things that seem important when you are facing death with someone who loves you.

The small hospital called their internal medicine specialist, who had trouble stopping the heart attack. The typical treatments only slowed the damage, and portions of my heart continued to die from lack of blood flow. Ralph spoke with Rick by phone as Rick was traveling to reach us, and the two of them discussed airlifting me to St. Louis for better care. Only one cardiologist practiced in the town, a doctor who was leaving for a month's vacation in India the next day, and we requested he be brought in. Rick arrived, and he and Ralph prayed for my healing.

The minute the cardiologist entered my room, he began to bark orders for changing my treatment. He will probably never win prizes for positive bedside manner, but we are very grateful that he stopped the progress of the heart attack before he left town. God answered our prayers through his expertise.

After alerting friends and family, Carey and Mark flew to St. Louis and arrived at the hospital later that same day. We spent the next week watching the green lines on my heart monitor screen together. I was delighted when I moved from the ICU to a regular room. Having Rick and the kids by my side was the best medicine I could have, and I finally got well enough to fly home. None of us ever wants to visit the St. Louis area again.

Home Again

We all started to relax when we got on the plane back to Michigan, but our relief lasted less than twenty-four hours. The next day I had a second heart attack. Rick broke the land-speed record rushing me to the University of Michigan Hospital, where the doctors tested me extensively and recommended a cardiac catheterization. I remember feeling strange watching the inside of my heart on a computer monitor.

The catheterization should have been a relatively routine test, but as one of my doctors said since then, "I've learned that if something can go wrong with your treatment, it probably will." I was allergic to the dye that they used to illuminate the arteries. Only minutes into the procedure, I developed enormous hives, and my entire body ballooned.

My eyes swelled shut, and I began to suffocate as my trachea closed. My arteries must be especially photogenic, because as I struggled for breath and the attending nurse reported my increasing symptoms, the doctor kept saying, "Just a few more pictures." Finally, at the insistence of the nurse, he gave the order to administer epinephrine to stop my allergic reaction. Then the staff discovered that they had no epinephrine in the procedure room. I thought to myself, "This is a really stupid way to die after all I've been through," and then panicked as the nurse ran to the next procedure room for the medicine. I was still gasping later when they wheeled my stretcher into the hall to wait for transport to my room. I squeaked out, "I can't breathe," but the staff member dismissed me with, "You're going to be fine," and left me there alone.

By the time I got back to my room, I looked like the Pillsbury Doughboy; I was so swollen that I could not move at all and could barely speak. My rheumatologist, Joseph McCune, came in, greeted me briefly, and left quickly. As he walked down the hall, I could hear him shouting, "What have you done to my patient?" I was delighted to be in his care since I could not speak for myself.

I recovered from the heart attacks and dye reaction in the hospital for three weeks and did very little for the rest of the summer. Dr. McCune and the outstanding cardiologist he had recommended for me, Dr. Rubenfire, determined together that my heart attacks were caused by vasculitis, a rare complication of lupus, a disease Dr. McCune had recently discovered I had. They decided to try a six-month course of a special chemotherapy regimen to put the lupus into remission.

From July through December, I went into the hospital for three days a month: one day of preparatory medicines, one day of infusion, and one day of recovery medicines and fluids. The nurses dressed in hazardous materials outfits to carry the poisons they were hooking up to my IV, and we joked about my glowing in the dark after treatments.

Rick and the kids spent most of the days with me, alternating visits. When we got tired of puzzles, we invented a game watching the cars at a stop sign outside my window. As the cars approached, we bet on which of them would stop completely, which would pause slightly, and which would just drive on through. My family and friends prayed for us. We did not completely foil the lupus, but I did not have any new heart symptoms for a year. At the time I did not realize that my adventures in the world of medicine had just begun.

Admitting J Was Sick

I can understand now why the St. Louis emergency room doctor hesitated to admit me. I had none of the ordinary risk factors for heart attack. I exercised and was not overweight, had never smoked, did not drink, was only forty-seven years old, and had low cholesterol levels. I lived on a diet of health food and had taken vitamins for decades. In fact, my daughter later quipped that the heart attacks must have been caused by a diet of broccoli and brown rice. But we had recently discovered that I had lupus, a disease that can attack the heart no matter how clean your living has been.

Until my forty-fifth year, I boasted that a bottle of Tylenol usually expired before I finished it. I did not have headaches, didn't allow myself to sleep in, and never missed work. I was raised in a family environment that had stoic tendencies, and we simply didn't give in to little things like illness. If we complained of aches and pains, my parents might say "Big deal!" or "Get over it." As a result, as an adult I often overlooked or ignored signs that my health was failing. Finally, however, my body would not let me ignore them.

When I was eighteen I began to have fainting spells, fevers, extreme exhaustion, and joint pain. I seemed to have a terrible, long-lasting case of the flu. My family doctor discovered that my white blood cell count was dangerously low and ordered me to bed. So I spent the winter of my senior year in high school resting, getting up only for meals, doctor's appointments, and blood tests that showed slow but steady progress. I felt lonely and sad to miss these last days of high school with my friends. My doctor finally succumbed to my begging him to allow me to begin college in the fall, but I became very ill in the first two months and had to drop out in October. I was so weak that I could barely walk through the administration building to complete the forms the university insisted I fill out in person.

Throughout my adult years I had similar flu-like periods. Doctors puzzled over the symptoms and never managed to name the disease. Rest, again, was the only suggested treatment. Eventually I would recover and return to my normal routine.

At age forty-six I could no longer ignore my body's symptoms. I remember waking up in the morning so tired that I cried to think of going to work. Every part of my body ached. Strange rashes appeared on my face. Spots appeared and disappeared in my mouth. I wondered if I had a tumor or brain disease because, when I was exhausted, I would do things like drop the car keys into the trash can while, with my other hand, I put the trash onto the kitchen counter. Finally, the swelling and pain in my joints became so bad that I could no longer write on the board or my students' papers in the college classes I was teaching. I took a leave of absence for a semester to rest and try to find out what was wrong with me.

I visited physical medicine and rehabilitation doctors, internal medicine specialists, dermatologists, and endocrinologists. They treated my symptoms but never really found the cause. One doctor with a particular lack of insight looked over my chart and said, "Mrs. Wallace, are you depressed? If I had all the problems you have, I'd be depressed." I had spent twenty years as a counselor and knew that my symptoms were not in my head. Her dismissal of my medical condition was ludicrous, and she later told me she was astonished when she heard I had lupus. Ironically, at the same time that I was struggling to help doctors understand what was happening to my body, I shared very little with family and friends about the intense pain that I was experiencing.

During my leave of absence, through a chance occurrence that some might label providence and some God, my neighbor Nancy noticed I was limping and asked me about it. I shared some of my story with Nancy, who had lupus, and she suggested that I might have lupus also. I had heard of this disease but knew nothing about it. Nancy recommended her doctor, Dr. Joseph McCune, who was expert in lupus and known for his diagnostic skills.

In September 1991 Rick and I met Dr. McCune and were finally on our way to learning why my health had fluctuated so wildly over the years. Nancy's hunch had been correct, and I did, indeed, have lupus.

Lupus, an autoimmune disease, causes the body's defense system to become hyperactive, attacking its own organs and tissues like it would attack a virus or bacteria. Typical symptoms include arthritis, exhaustion, kidney failure, skin rashes, inflammation of the lungs or heart, blood clots, and neurologic disorders, but those of us who live with it have learned that lupus can do whatever it decides to do whenever it decides to do it. We learn to live with daily pain and exhaustion and to cope with what seem to be an endless succession of major and minor medical complications. More than one million Americans live with lupus, and the five-year survival rate has soared from fifty percent in 1955 to about ninety percent today due to new treatments. There is no cure for lupus, and those of us who have it will ultimately die of it or from the medicines we take to control our symptoms.

Strange as it seems, I felt relieved at discovering this. I now know this is a common response. Many of the chronically ill have wandered around the medical world being poked and prodded and not helped for so long that they feel good having their disease defined, even if the diagnosis frightens them.

Now I could read about my enemy and learn the best ways to fight it. Now I could stop looking for the answer to *what* and start learning *how*. As the battle began, I could plan my campaign. I have had many ups and downs in my battle for health during the years that followed my diagnosis, and I have learned much about how to win the skirmishes that I would like to share with you.

I did not live happily ever after with no headaches. In fact, my physical health has continued to deteriorate in many ways. Dr. McCune prescribed medicines to control my symptoms, and by spring of 1992, shortly before my first heart attack, I was walking up stairs at a normal pace, rather than with two feet on each step and dragging myself with my arms on the railing. I could get up in the morning without crying. I felt very encouraged. Unfortunately, however, the stress of the lupus added to the stress of the full-time work I was doing at the time had combined to cause the heart attack in St. Louis.

The Saga Continues

After my first two heart attacks and the chemotherapy, I recovered but still did not feel well. In January 1993 we discovered that my gall bladder was severely diseased, and my surgeon removed it in February. This surgery seemed like an answer to prayer because it was relatively easy to handle compared to heart attacks, dye reactions, and chemotherapy.

Yet I continued to have persistent chest pain. Further testing showed a small spot on my lung. Dr. McCune explained that lupus patients often have lung infections and ordered a needle biopsy of the spot. He was leaving town the next day to present a paper at a national conference and, in his typical thoughtful way, had arranged for a pathologist to review the biopsy immediately so that he could arrange my treatment before he left.

We were all amazed by the result: with tears in his eyes, Dr. McCune came to the post-op room and told us that I had large-cell lung cancer. We had begun to understand the enemy we faced in lupus, but we were completely unprepared to fight a battle against cancer at the same time. Within minutes we all had tears in our eyes. For days afterwards I would begin to cry spontaneously, angry that this invader was growing in my body. Wasn't having lupus and heart disease enough for one family to handle?

I still don't know how he did it, but before he left that day, Dr. McCune arranged for further testing as well as for me to meet with a pulmonologist, who read the tests, told us that my tumor seemed to be contained, and suggested that I had a good chance of recovery. Within days I met with the thoracic surgeon who would later remove my left lung. Because of my two recent heart attacks and gall bladder surgery, the doctors agreed that I still needed a few weeks to heal before this next major operation. This wait provided a challenge for me: to know that I had cancer and do nothing to stop it for some weeks forced me to rely on my belief that God's timing is always perfect, no matter what it may seem at the moment.

On the last day of March 1993, the surgeon removed the large lobe of my left lung, and I began the long and painful process of rehabilitation. The therapist came into my room the day after surgery with a device I was supposed to blow into to build up my remaining lung. She said, "This will hurt unbelievably, and you will not want to do it. But if you don't, you will never regain your ability to breathe well." Somehow her honesty helped me to do what I needed to do, often with tears running down my face, and recover as fully as I could. When not exercising I would lie as still as possible and pray for the days to pass quickly, knowing that it was only a matter of time before my body healed.

As hard as this was for me, I truly believe it was more difficult for my family, having to see me in pain with every movement and unable to do anything to stop it. The positive prognosis lifted our spirits: the surgeon removed all of the tumor and surrounding tissue and found no cancer in any of my lymph nodes! I remain free of lung cancer seventeen years later, thank God. Every year I bake a cake for the surgeon, Dr. Orringer, and his staff to celebrate my lung-cancer-free anniversary.

As my lung healed, my doctors expected that all of the pain in my chest would disappear, but it didn't. So they scheduled a colonoscopy. In June 1993 a wonderful gastroenterologist, Kimberly Brown, found a large tumor in my colon. Dr. Brown told me that more surgery would be required. Again, the operation was postponed until I had sufficiently healed from the surgery on my lung.

In August 1993, Dr. Eckhauser successfully removed the tumor and eighteen inches of my colon. The day of my discharge, Rick had to be out of town for a conference, so the kids came to pick me up. After waiting together all morning for my paperwork to be processed, Carey gathered my belongings and Mark went to retrieve the car. As Carey wheeled me out into the hallway, I began to have chest pains. I wanted to go home anyway, but Carey refused to budge. I reluctantly returned to the desk clerk and told her I was having chest pains. Without looking up from her paperwork, she replied, "All of the doctors are at lunch right now."

Carey was furious. I almost started laughing at the absurdity of the situation. Who has a heart attack in a wheelchair on the way *out* of the hospital? I wouldn't have believed it myself except that it was happening to me. But by this time the chest pains were severe and too familiar. I calmly asked the desk clerk to page a doctor immediately.

The doctors who had taken care of me for ten days had officially discharged me moments before. So a cardiology resident who had never met me responded to the page. The resident was a poor listener, pompous, and overbearing. He seemed more upset about this interruption to his day than he was about my symptoms. "I am confident," he said, "that you are not having a heart attack."

By this time, I not only had chest pain but the classic electrical impulses down both arms that I had experienced before. I was absolutely confident that I *was* having a heart attack. I had been perfectly calm, assuming that the doctor would treat me appropriately and stop this heart attack. When he dismissed my symptoms instead, I became insistent. "I am not going to lie here in front of my children and die needlessly," I said. "You will begin IV nitroglycerin on me immediately, or I may create a real problem." To keep me quiet, the resident hooked me up to a nitroglycerin IV and ordered the heart enzyme tests. When the tests came back several hours later, they showed a significant heart attack in progress.

Once again Rick rushed to the hospital and informed Dr. Eckhauser's team about my heart attack and the resident's response. Dr. Eckhauser's team, who knew me well, arranged for me to be placed back in their care in the surgical ICU. They stopped the progress of the heart attack, and I slowly recovered.

The next day, when my cardiologist visited me in the ICU, I told him about my experience with the resident, and he was incredulous. "What did he think was happening?" he asked. He forced the cardiology resident to come to my room and apologize for his behavior. But his audacious apology consisted of telling me, "I would have bet my medical license that you were not having a heart attack."

"If you had done that," I responded, "you wouldn't be practicing medicine today." Dr. Rubenfire also wrote me a prescription to carry with me at all times: "Mrs. Wallace is subject to MI caused by vasospastic spasm. She responds well to IV nitroglycerin and should be started on this as soon as possible." Showing this prescription to emergency room doctors has helped to save my life during four subsequent heart attacks.

The overwhelming majority of physicians who have treated me have been both caring and competent. Occasionally, however, I have found doctors whose egos have outstripped their common sense. I could understand the emergency room doctor not catching my heart problem, since the only risk factor I had was lupus, but only arrogance explains a doctor who will not listen to a patient who has already lived through two heart attacks and knows what they feel like. When we encounter this arrogance or lack of understanding, we must stand up to it and insist on the treatment we need. In chapter six I will discuss ways to develop relationships with physicians so that you can work together at doing well.

What I Learned

At first I was angry at the cardiac resident's carelessness and other mistakes people have made in my care over the years. But I have learned to let these situations go and use them for good. The first step in this process was to recognize God's grace toward my own errors and extend it to others. David, a man after God's own heart, also was a man who needed forgiveness. He reminds us of this great truth in Psalm 103:

> *He will not always accuse,*
> *   nor will he harbor his anger forever;*
> *he does not treat us as our sins deserve*
> *   or repay us according to our iniquities.*

> *For ... as far as the east is from the west,*
> *   so far has he removed our transgressions from us*
> *   (vv. 9–10, 12).*

Most medical personnel work extremely hard to keep us as healthy as possible. But they all make mistakes along the way, and we need to forgive them. When I think of myself daily as a sinner in need of grace, I have impetus to forgive others, no matter what the sin. Thank God I have never caused another person's death or disability, but I know that I might have. Realizing this humbles me and saves me from the constant, draining pain of anger and seeking for vengeance. When I give up the anger, I gain energy to do what God wants me to be doing with the additional days He has given me.

Second, God has blessed me with the knowledge that nothing that happens to me is beyond His control. I can trust that if it would be better for me in the long run not to experience something, God's power can accomplish this. I am in His hand and am loved by Him, no matter what. The circumstances in which I find myself afford me opportunities to trust in Him, to learn about Him, and to grow to be more in character like Him. With the psalmist, I can honestly say, "It was good for me to be afflicted so that I might learn your decrees" (119:71), and "I know, O Lord, that your laws are righteous, and in faithfulness you have afflicted me. May your unfailing love be my comfort, according to your promise to your servant" (Psalm 119:75–76).

Third, I have learned that God has a new task for me. Part of my job now is to help people who live with chronic illness and their loved ones to learn from their experiences. Although my illness prevents me from working outside of my home, I find that God continues to give me assignments. After a lifetime of good health, a neighbor needs counsel when doctors discover cancer. A friend asks me to speak with someone who is still struggling to find a diagnosis for a set of symptoms. A pastor refers a couple having difficulty relating to the elephant in the living room that is sickness. A medical student wants to know how to become a really good doctor. God has uniquely fitted me, by academic and professional background as well as through some of my most difficult life experiences, to help these people. I praise Him for providing this work for me and help for them.

Accepting Your Situation

Why is it so difficult for us to accept that we have an illness that is affecting our lives? For me the first barrier was my irrational self-confidence. I had always felt independent, especially before I put my faith in God. My first line of defense was to ignore what was going on: if I didn't talk about it, maybe it wouldn't exist.

Two heart attacks in eight days smashed this myth, and I moved to a second stage in which I accepted the fact that my body had a problem, but I believed I could eliminate that problem with diet, exercise, and medicine. If I could fix what I was now forced to admit was going on in my body, then I could begin again to ignore it and continue to achieve my various agendas. I approached this just as I would approach a problem at work or home: rational behavior coupled with my tenacity would take care of this annoyance.

In all of life's difficult situations, God often allows us to stew in these stages until we are ready to accept the fact that He has been in control all of the time. My lupus did not surprise God. All along He has been much more interested in my spiritual growth than in my physical healing. I have had a great deal to learn, and He took the time to teach me because of His deep love for me. What happened next shows the process of teaching and learning about gratitude, relying on God, living with pain, changing life attitudes, and finding strength and hope in the midst of difficulties.

What Does It All Mean?

My body no longer works as well as it did seventeen years ago. In the two-year period I have just described, I was diagnosed with lupus, heart disease, gall bladder disease, lung cancer, and colon cancer. Since that time, I have had or still have:

- bladder cancer
- sclerotic mesenteritis
- trigeminal neuralgia
- peripheral neuropathy
- debilitating arthritis
- chronic spinal disc problems
- numerous tendon and muscle tears
- loss of balance due to inner ear damage
- double vision
- Sjogren's syndrome
- gastroparesis
- GERD
- esophageal spasm and erosions
- endomitosis
- bursitis in hips, knees, and shoulders
- Plantar fascitis
- Morton's neuromas
- de Quervain's syndrome
- tendinitis
- repeated skin cancers requiring surgeries
- asthma
- a host of other maladies

The last time an intern finished taking my history, I told him that I was really just a test patient who was there to see if he was gullible enough to believe my story. When I lay it out sickness by sickness, I am overwhelmed myself. But I continue to live through new unexpected diagnoses and have learned to do well at being chronically ill while coping with acute illness when it arises.

Rick likes to point out that God wants us to love Him with all our heart, soul, mind, and body. These illnesses have affected only my body; my heart, soul, and mind are still readily available for loving God. Since loving Him and His other children remains our major task here on earth, I am still in good shape. I rejoice in being able to carry out this assignment. Even at times when I am not able to walk or care for myself physically, I can pray for others in confidence that my heavenly Father listens and hears.

In addition to this blessing, I am able to participate remarkably fully in the world most of the time. I can walk by myself, sometimes with a cane. Most days I still cook, play the piano, and use a computer. I watched my children graduate from high school, college, and graduate school. I occasionally have the energy to attend concerts to watch them play music. Our small Bible study group meets weekly at our house, and I usually make it to church. I love to bake and send treats to friends, family, and Rick's students. I talk to friends and family daily. People love me, and I love them.

I spend a lot of time hanging out at hospitals and doctors' offices and often see people who struggle with much more difficult physical problems than mine. I do not have diabetes or liver disease or kidney failure or congestive heart failure. My lungs function remarkably well, considering my struggles with lung cancer. I have so much to be thankful for!

I am a person who has illnesses, but illnesses do not define me. God defined me before I was born. My life is full of fun, and yours can be as well, whether you are a person facing illness or the loving caregiver of a person facing illness. I hope to use my experiences to teach you about navigating the healthcare system, managing family and friendship relationships, living a "healthy" life, and growing your relationship with God through the adversity of illness. My prayer is that *my* story will help you make *your* story more joyful.

In Summary

1. Often we know that something is wrong before the professionals can name it. Keep asking questions until they can, and learn to insist on the care you need.

2. Keep alert, but do not let new challenges sink you.

3. Use your bad experiences with medical situations to grow in knowledge of your body's needs and in reliance on God's plan.

4. Learn to thank God for what you don't have as well as for what you do have.

5. Believe that you can do well at living with sickness.

Chapter Two

~

Developing an Attitude
of Gratitude

<u>*You will learn:*</u>

- to find the joy in every circumstance
- to serve the world instead of feeling sorry for yourself
- to use your gifts and time wisely

Take my life and let it be
Consecrated, Lord, to Thee;
Take my moments and my days
Let them flow in ceaseless praise.

FRANCES RIDLEY HAVERGAL

~

*I*n fifteen months I had experienced three heart attacks, anaphylactic shock, lung cancer, gall bladder disease, colon cancer, three surgeries, and six rounds of in-patient chemotherapy. I still battled the lupus and was continually exhausted. Each time I returned home from the hospital, I measured my progress by my daily walks: first past one house, then two houses, then to the corner and back, and, finally, around the block.

But I was still alive! I could love my husband, children, and friends. I could do some work around the house. I could help others by listening to them and pray for those I cared about. My understanding of God's will has matured as I experience illness and watch others cope with physical challenges, and I am grateful for my life.

Faith in the Midst of Despair

This growth in faith began with an experience involving my daughter. Carey was fourteen, we had just moved from Georgia to Michigan, and she was a few weeks into high school when we discovered that she needed a complicated surgery. For several years she had been treated for debilitating scoliosis. The curve in her spine had progressed to 82 degrees and was crushing her lungs and other organs. We took her to the Mayo Clinic in Rochester, Minnesota, where a well-known surgeon scheduled an eight-hour operation that would fuse all of her vertebrae and install two metal rods in her back to partially straighten her spine.

Carey and I arrived for tests three days before the surgery and settled into a house that had been created for the families of children being treated at Mayo. We both felt frightened and a little sorry for ourselves. I was unhappy that she had to face major surgery at such a young age and experience the pain that we knew was coming.

Ten families filled the house to capacity. Parents and siblings of the patients stayed there full-time. Patients spent most of their days at the hospital but sometimes had passes to stay for a day or two with their families between treatments. Most had life-threatening illnesses; many had cancer. Uniformly, the parents' faces reflected fear, resignation, watchfulness, and anxiety. The siblings seemed confused and lonely. The children being treated had tattoos on their heads to guide their radiation treatments, surgical scars on their bodies, and missing legs and arms. They also had irrepressible smiles. These children were treated by a medical team that never gave up on them, and they had learned to never give up themselves. They were all fighters.

Spending two weeks with these families transformed the way I thought about Carey's situation; I began to develop an attitude of gratitude. If the surgery went well and she was not paralyzed, Carey would get better. She would have some lasting effects from this disease but would live and have a fairly normal life. I was blessed. I developed compassion for these other families that I could not have experienced before living with them. I also formed a great admiration for the way they continued on in the face of daunting odds and difficult times. I began to realize what faith meant: not knowing but believing.

I believe that watching those with illness choose hope rather than despair inspires the caring people of Rochester, Minnesota, the kindest city I have ever visited. Everyone, from the waitresses to the taxicab drivers, seemed to have an inordinate ability to express caring for others. People I had never met before and would never see again went out of their way to make me comfortable. The vulnerability of these very ill patients and their families brought out the best in the staff at the hospital; I have never been treated so well.

Living with these families at Mayo taught me that our attitude determines the direction of our lives, no matter what we face. We can bemoan our cancer or be glad that it is treatable. We can complain about our pain or be grateful that we have the use of all of our painful limbs. We can *always* find something for which to be thankful. On our wall hangs a sampler that I stitched years ago to remind myself:

> *Contentment is not the fulfillment of what you want,*
> *but the realization of what you already have.*

Getting Out of Ourselves

During my first heart attack in that small Missouri hospital, the staff placed me in an intensive care unit. Although medication had dulled some of the pain, my heart attack continued through the night. I was tired, worried, and lonely. When a nurse came to see me, I asked her to bring me something. Today I don't even remember what it was.

Anyone who has spent time in an ICU knows that the "rooms" are separated only by curtains so that staff can access a large number of very sick people quickly. Shortly after the nurse visited me, an ambulance brought in a man who had drowned and been resuscitated. His breathing sounded like Darth Vader punctuated with bouts of noisy and unpleasant gagging. All night the staff worked hard to monitor his machines and keep him breathing regularly. I began to be unhappy. Why didn't the nurse bring me what I had asked for? Why were they spending all of their energy on this man? What about ME?

Almost immediately God spoke to me. "This is just like you, Wendy, always thinking of yourself first. Has it occurred to you that this man and the staff need your prayers right now?" As usual, God was right. I began to pray for all of them: for strength, for wisdom, for the man's family, for the right decisions to be made. And I forgot about my petty concerns. I was grateful that the staff thought I was well enough to leave me alone for a few minutes. I was grateful that I was surviving a heart attack. I was grateful that God was still talking to me even though I was so selfish. My spirit grew calm, and I felt much better.

Later, the nurse did come to check on me. I asked how the man was doing and told her that I had been praying for all of them. She began to cry and thank me. She had been working for almost twenty hours and was both exhausted and discouraged. This small hospital rarely had so many crises at once, and the stresses of a long day had overwhelmed her. She also shared that God had been prodding her in many ways to go back to church and begin reading her Bible again and that she had put Him off because of her busy schedule. She saw my praying for her as another plea from God and decided to immediately renew her faith commitment.

God frequently reminds me to enjoy the blessings He has given me rather than to complain about my situation. For example, for many months a degenerated disc in my back created such intense pain that I could not drive. I had always taken for granted that if I needed something from the store, I could hop into the car and get it. I assumed that if I wanted to visit my father in his assisted living facility, I could. Through prayer, time, and good medical care, my disc has now healed enough to allow me to drive short distances. Last week I drove the two miles to the market for the first time and was excited—as I should always have been—just to be getting groceries! Concentrating on how God has blessed me brings me great joy.

Joy from Pain

As hard as it is to believe, I would not trade my experience for another life. Before I was ill, I took my days for granted and often used them carelessly. I could spend hours obsessing over getting everything just right for a family gathering. I spent precious energy being angry with people for offenses they had committed against me. I might put off phone calls to friends or family indefinitely if I had *important work* to do.

Today I see every hour as a gift. Because of my situation, I am much more aware than most people of the fragility of life. Before I get out of bed each morning, I thank God for another day, ask His direction in using the time He has given me, and pray that I will reflect His light to everyone I meet. This prayer puts life in perspective for me: God has blessed me with life, and I should use that life as well as I can for His glory.

No longer do I waste my time (and God's) in over-cleaning a house for guests. No longer do I waste the little energy I have in staying angry with someone else. No longer will I put off a conversation in order to accomplish something that the world might see as more important than an encounter specially put into my day by God.

This awareness of the preciousness of life has transformed our entire family. We appreciate one another much more. Never does a phone call end without an "I love you" on both ends of the line. Rarely do we get angry at one another. Hardly ever does a disagreement last for more than a few minutes, even though we love a hearty debate over almost any issue. (We especially love to argue about things that we don't really have any facts about.)

Our church observes a College Student Sunday, when returning students lead the worship service. During the first year of physical turmoil for me, Carey was asked to present the sermon, and she chose as her scripture Isaiah 55:12:

> *You will go out in joy*
> *and be led forth in peace;*
> *the mountains and hills*
> *will burst into song before you,*
> *and all the trees of the field*
> *will clap their hands.*

Carey talked about what our family had gone through. Her bottom line was that God had blessed us through difficulties and was leading us into joy and peace. We were listening to the song of the mountains and hills, and the trees of the field were clapping their hands for us. She challenged the congregation to make specific commitments toward God's plan for their lives, even supplying paper and envelopes for them to write down their commitment so that she could mail it to them in six months' time for their review.

We do not deny at all that great pain and suffering accompany illness. I know that Carey would never have chosen for me to be very sick for almost half of her life. But clearly we have all learned that every day, whether pain-filled or pain-free, should be used wisely. She noted well that the atmosphere in our home was more caring, tender, and focused on what was really important. As she stated in her sermon, "It is difficult to worry about dirty socks in the face of mortality."

If I could, I would tell this to everyone I come in contact with every day. I am not sure that it is learnable except through experience, but it certainly is one of the most important things that I know. When I see people upset about waiting in a line of traffic, worried about a situation at work, or angry at some real or imagined slight from another person, I want to shake them and say, "It is not important. Look at the wonder of your life. Love your friends and family unreservedly. Spend time with God. Use your minutes wisely."

God has designed life so that we can find joy through pain. Walking through the valleys fits us to enjoy the view from the mountaintop. The Bible is full of examples of this, from Abraham to Job. The Psalms speak of indescribable betrayal and agony as well as of delight and joy, as many of them predict the crucifixion and resurrection of Jesus Christ.

Modern people want pain to disappear. Of course pain medicines and treatments have an important part in alleviating suffering caused by illness, and many of us with chronic illnesses would not function well without them. However, we often try to eliminate even the appearance of suffering in our advanced society. This attitude cuts us off from experiencing joy at the highest level because it denies the basic truth that life on earth will always be incomplete.

I urge you, as you confront your illness or that of a loved one, to accept pain as a part of your life. Make it your teacher. Use it to come to the realization of how much you have. Live through it to reach the highest joy you can imagine.

Why Am I Still Here?

Years ago we lived in a small town near a wonderful greenhouse called Glei's. Glei's began as a roadside stand run by Carl Glei, a local farmer with a small orchard. Over the years the greenhouse grew into a sizeable business, serving the entire county and trucking produce into the large city several hours away. Mr. Glei's sons took over as he aged, but he continued to work every day, arriving as soon as he came home from daily Mass. When he was in his nineties, he was unable to work in the greenhouses or fields, but he continued to gift-wrap the many houseplants they sold. Mr. Glei offered gardening advice to anyone who would stop to ask him a question about varieties of roses, pest control, fertilizing, times for planting, or anything else having to do with growing things.

One day after asking his advice, I told him how much I admired and respected him and hoped to be working when I was his age. He shared something with me that I will never forget. "Some of my friends say to me, 'I don't know why I don't just die and go to heaven, I'm so old and useless.' And I say to them, 'You are here because the Lord still has something for you to do. So get off your rear end and do it!'"

I believed him then, and I believe him now. I have found, even during weeks and months in which I am confined to hospital, home, or bed, that the Lord still has things for me to do. I could spend those weeks bemoaning the fact that I can no longer do what I used to do, or I could spend them accepting the assignments He has for me in my new state of circumstances. I am grateful to God for life and for developing in me an attitude of gratitude rather than of anger.

Using God's Gifts as We Are Able

Rick and I have a good friend whom we have known for over forty years who struggles with an inherited illness that has gradually reduced his mobility. George has always loved children. Although he has never had any children of his own, his nieces and nephews, godchildren, neighbors, and children of friends all love him.

Forced to retire from his work as a chemist because of his illness, George immediately began to volunteer at the local hospital, spending time with babies who are hospitalized for extended periods of time. George's love for these babies is evident to their parents, which takes pressure off of them to be with their child every moment. His is truly a labor of love, but he would be the first to tell you that he receives more from his ministry than he gives.

George's life revolves around "his" babies. He schedules his own medical appointments, arranges his transportation, and changes his sleeping patterns according to their needs. He is a man of deep faith, and he would certainly state that his primary goal is to serve God. But loving the babies and their families remains his most important task, the one on which he spends his limited energy. Instead of feeling sorry for himself, George experiences great joy in blessing these little ones.

Becoming a Grateful Saint

We all know people who are constantly unhappy regardless of their circumstances. Some of us are blessed to know those who are always happy regardless of their circumstances. My experience has shown me that the difference between these people is usually a strong faith in God.

In *The Saints among Us,* George Gallup, Jr. studied the lives of those he described as saints in today's society. Rather than being specially gifted in terms of wealth, education, or status, Gallup's saints were overwhelmingly poor African American women with a strong faith in the Lord. They had learned the secret Paul speaks of in Philippians 4. After encouraging his brothers and sisters in Christ to "Rejoice in the Lord always" and think about whatever is true, noble, right, pure, lovely, admirable, excellent, or praiseworthy, he sums up his stance by declaring, "I can do everything through him who gives me strength" (vv. 4, 8, 13).

The women Gallup studied endured hardships due to their poverty, race, and gender; life in this world was not fair to them. But rather than becoming bitter, they became more faithful. Rather than focusing on their pain, they relied on God for strength and joy and received both.

Chronic illness is not fair; when you consider carefully, you find that there are many aspects of life that are unfair. But chronic illness can lead to chronic peace if you let God guide you through it. I have seen lives eaten up by the question, "Why did this happen to me?" God has taught me that I might just as well ask Him, "Why was I blessed with such a wonderful family, a good education, a free country in which to live, more food than I should eat, and a saving knowledge of you?" We will not know the answers to these questions until we reach heaven, but we can know the attitude with which we should approach all the days He has given us here on earth until then: an attitude of gratitude.

In Summary

1. In every situation in which we find ourselves, there is always something to be thankful for. Look for it.

2. When you begin to feel self-pity, get out of yourself and serve the rest of the world however you can.

3. Find the joy in your circumstances.

4. Do not waste time in being upset.

5. Use the gifts God has given you.

6. Learn to rely on the Lord in order to develop a lasting attitude of gratitude.

Chapter Three

~

Our Being Sick Affects Our Families

You will learn:

- to have difficult discussions with your loved ones
- to care for your caregivers
- to prioritize quality family time
- to deepen your friendship with God

*Resolved... That I will live
so as I shall wish I had done
when I come to die.*

JONATHAN EDWARDS

Recently I overheard my son Mark tell a friend that whenever his phone rings he wonders momentarily if this is the call telling him that I have died. This is not an unwarranted fear. Seven times Mark has either been called to emergency rooms or taken me there when I have had a heart attack, and he knows that statistically one-third of heart attack patients do not survive. I understood his comment, and my heart cried for him.

As a wife and mother, my first concern when diagnosed with a life-threatening illness was for my family. Carey was seventeen and Mark fourteen when I first learned I had lupus. They were eighteen and fifteen when I had my first two heart attacks. In my weakest moments, I worry about what they all will do without me when I die. Rick hasn't taken care of paying the bills in years and doesn't remember to make his skin cancer check-up appointments. I worry about becoming a burden to them and fear their resentment over having to take care of a sick mother and wife. I worry that my illness or death will scar them for life. I worry that dealing with this at such young ages will damage the kids' faith in God. And I know that they worry about me as well.

I don't like to admit that I worry my family. When I get up from a not-so-good night's sleep and look terrible, I see the concern in their eyes. If they phone and my voice is not strong, they ask "Are you really okay?" When I grimace suddenly, take a nitroglycerin tablet to suppress a heart pain, or admit that I'm not feeling well enough to take a walk, they are reminded that my body is deteriorating and in pain. I hate worrying them, but I cannot change that.

The Full Disclosure Contract

One thing I have done to assuage the worry is to make a full disclosure agreement with my family: I have agreed never to keep medical secrets from them. When I have information, they receive the information. Usually I try to be dispassionate when I tell them the results of tests, diagnoses, and possibilities of treatment. After they have had a chance to ask questions, we can discuss options together.

This has been a valuable policy. Even when Carey and Mark were six hundred miles away at college, they knew that they did not have to see me physically to be able to know that I was telling them the whole truth about my condition. We can all deal most easily with that which is known; the unknown is much more frightening.

Obviously, for younger children you must choose carefully how and to what extent to explain your illness according to their ability to understand. But you should be honest even with small children and not underestimate what they already know or are guessing. One of our friends assured his preteen son that he would beat the cancer that was ravaging his body. When our friend later died of the cancer, his son felt both grief at his loss and anger at his father for betraying his trust. If our friend had been both positive about fighting the cancer *and* honest about possible outcomes, his son would have had time to grieve with his dad's support.

This is a gift that you can give to those you love: tell them that you will always tell them. Promise not to suffer in silence. Agree to pull the weight of knowledge together, with love. The energy that they would have expended being anxious about whether they know the truth should be channeled into helping you make good medical decisions based on the information you have all shared.

At the same time, it is important that you not make your children your confidants. They should know the medical facts; they do not necessarily need to know every time you are feeling discouraged or that your aches and pains are particularly acute one day. You should never lie to them about your condition, but neither should you continually put them in the position of being told that their parent, whom they love, has pain that nobody can control.

In practice this means that you should tell them that you would rather not go to the baseball game with them because the ride in the car and sitting in hard bleacher seats does not sound like a good idea that day. You should not call your children in the morning to tell them that you are having trouble convincing yourself to get out of bed because of pain. In other words, be forthcoming when your condition affects your family and their decisions, but do not share every challenge. These struggles should be shared with your spouse and adult friends.

Difficult Conversations

Before one particularly risky surgery, when Carey and Mark were eighteen and fifteen, our family sat down to plan my funeral. Carey later wrote a short story for a college freshman writing class about this bizarre dinnertime conversation that affected all of us profoundly. Mostly factual, the story shows some of the ways in which real people cope with real pain. (See her story, "Stand on Your Porch and Scream," at the end of this chapter.)

We talked about funerals in general. Carey didn't want flowers because she loves flowers and didn't want them spoiled for her by my funeral. She also didn't want visitation, because she didn't want to stand around talking to people she doesn't really know. Mark pushed food around his plate and said little. We discussed embalming and cemeteries. We even talked about music and preachers. All of us cried.

At the time, I thought of our discussion as a practical exercise we approached together. Later I realized that this conversation was a gift I had been able to give to my family. Although our ideas about funerals have changed since that day, the process strengthened our family. Grieving my death will be difficult for them. By encouraging them to do some anticipatory grieving, I could comfort them in person as they considered this inevitable event. Together we looked at the practical aspects of funerals, but beyond that we admitted that one day they would be living in this world without me. I know now that my family will make it through my death and thrive after I am gone. In some ways, in fact, I think discussing my death enabled us to face the fact that each of us will leave the others at some point in time when we leave this earth.

Being Sick Affects Our Marriage Relationships

Rick and I met when we were students at the University of Michigan and got married six months later against the advice of our parents. We were twenty-one years old, very much in love, and sure we knew what we were doing. Our early marriage had its ups and downs, full of passion and caring as well as hurt and adjustment. We moved to Pennsylvania for jobs and then to Connecticut for graduate school.

When I became pregnant with Carey eight years later, we were delighted. But Carey's birth forced us for the first time to confront our mortality. Her face-upward position and large size stalled her delivery, and when she went into distress the doctors did an emergency cesarean section that resulted in unexpected complications. Rick faced the prospect of losing me while sitting alone on the floor of the corridor outside the surgery room at 4 a.m. He still tears up when he talks about that night.

As a child, Rick attended church every week with his parents. My family did not attend church, but I read the entire Bible at age thirteen and became convinced of its truth. After we married, we attended church regularly. Everywhere we lived, we became involved in church life, often serving as leaders of youth groups and Sunday school teachers. We were educated, "good" people. Both of us tried to follow the teachings of Jesus.

But neither of us wanted to admit that we did not control our own destinies, so neither of us had totally surrendered control of our lives to the Lord. As I was praying during a difficult bump in my road, I admitted to God that I was powerless to deal with my life. I committed to trust Him from then on because I knew that He loved me and wanted the best for me. Rather than reacting to what was or was not happening in my life, I would truly live out the reality that His grace is sufficient for me. I could now honestly say with David, "I trust in you, O Lord; I say, 'You are my God.' My times are in your hands" (Psalm 31:14–15).

I kept this decision private, but God's blessing of it turned my life around. My transformation astounded Rick; I looked like his wife, but I didn't always act like her. My anxiety and desire to control my and my family's life all but vanished. As I look back, I realize I had spent the first years of my Christian life trying to do good things in imitation of Christ because of God's graciousness toward me. When I came to the end of myself, I realized that God wanted me to learn more about Him and trust Him at a deeper level.

Later Rick had an encounter with a godly friend who led him to a similar prayer. When he came home and excitedly shared the peace that he had found as a result of this prayer, I told him what had happened between God and me ten months earlier, and we rejoiced together. That day marked the beginning of a closeness that we had never experienced before, despite the bond of love we had shared for years. This has since affected everything in our lives, including our daily prayers and devotions, parenting, decision-making, and use of money.

By bringing us both to His throne of grace and helping us understand His love for us and how to share it, God set the stage for us to handle my illness in the subsequent years.

I truly believe that if we had not experienced God's grace previously, we would not have known how to draw upon and trust in it through the painful times we have lived through.

Without God our marriage would probably have dissolved. The divorce rate among couples dealing with chronic illness is astronomical. Without Rick's love and care, I would probably have died by now. I have asked him to share what it is like to be the spouse of someone who is chronically ill and how he copes with this through God's power and grace.

Being the Partner of a Chronically Ill Person: Rick's Thoughts

When we met, Wendy seemed unusually vigorous and healthy. I had never met anyone with her energy. She juggled an enormous class load, worked in the theater program, volunteered service, and held two part-time jobs to pay for her schooling. Her beauty, sense of humor, and energy attracted me.

Once we started dating seriously, she told me that she had been ill her freshman year in college and that the doctors had never determined the cause. She was so vibrant that I really didn't believe it. How could someone so full of life be sick? But her voice conveyed an intense concern that I had not heard before. Now when Wendy's illnesses trouble us, she reminds me that she warned me she was sick before I asked her to marry me, so I can't complain now!

Scripture tells us that the two become one when they marry. When Wendy became ill, in a sense I developed a chronic illness also. This illness that we share has brought limitations, unusual expenditures of energy and money, and uncertainty as well as joy.

Among the sorrows for me are watching Wendy live in pain and lose the ability to do things she once enjoyed. During the first ten years of our married life we traveled every summer, driving as far as Montreal or Nova Scotia. Even after the kids were born we regularly rented a small cottage on Cape Cod. During the past ten years, we have not traveled more than 150 miles from the University of Michigan Hospital. Before we leave on any trip, we check and re-check medications. I often must leave Wendy behind as I travel or participate in activities her body cannot tolerate.

Even when we were poor college students Wendy and I loved to entertain friends and family. For most of our kids' growing-up years, a typical Sunday afternoon included anywhere from one to ten random friends joining us to share a meal, play games, make music, or sit around talking. Today we entertain less, few visits last more than two hours, and Wendy may need to retire to her room to rest. She loves her friends and will wear herself out talking with them before they even know she is tired.

We also face the likelihood that she will not be alive for the weddings of our kids, the births of grandchildren, and other celebrations. In fact Wendy, who enjoys creating things for others with her hands, has started filling a "hope chest" of quilts and afghans for her as yet unborn grandchildren in case she is not here to make them later.

Yet Wendy's illness has also brought joy. Having faced the reality of a shortened life expectancy and the possibility of a sudden death has helped us to focus on what really matters. The pace of our lives has slowed, and we have come to cherish simple things, making more time for walks and talks and less time for fancy or complicated activities.

Praying together at the beginning and end of each day keeps us focused on what is important. For the past twenty-five years we have tried to take a half-hour walk together every day, time uninterrupted by children, telephones, or people stopping by. Wendy cannot always take a walk outside, but we try every day to at least sit or lie down together for half an hour of one-on-one time. We also spend at least one evening a week together without company or television. When her hands aren't too sore, we love to play old show tunes and jazz together, Wendy on piano and me on trombone.

Wendy's illness has also taught me to prioritize my work. At Wendy's urging we began to share housework early in our married life, and my ability to cook, clean, and do laundry has proved invaluable. She continues to organize the household and do most of the everyday work, but we are blessed that we can both fill most of the functions of running our family. For example, when Wendy needed to finish a draft of this book, I acted as her "wife" for a few days, just as she has done for me many times over the years when I faced a pressing deadline on a project, releasing her from meal preparation and daily chores while she spent time at the computer.

I find strength for being Wendy's partner through the grace of God. I am more likely now to seek His help, to recognize it when it comes, and to follow His lead when a crisis occurs. My individual prayer and study time in the mornings leads me to rely on God's grace, the greatest blessing in this world.

I am also strengthened through a special group of believers who meet weekly in our home to share our journeys and study the Bible together. These friends pray for us regularly and support us in tangible ways as well, bringing meals, providing rides to appointments, weeding gardens, buying groceries, sharing homemade foods, and showing God's love to us in thousands of small gestures. The fact that they come to our house for worship and study has often meant that Wendy is able to "do church" on days when she cannot leave home to attend our church's regular service. One good friend from the group walks with me once a week, providing opportunity for us to share our struggles and encourage one another to grow as husbands and dads.

I believe Wendy is alive today because of the faithful prayers of many believers. I would not have been able to persevere without praying friends who understand my life situation and care for us. Having people ask me how I am doing and really wanting to know the answer means a great deal to me; having them actually pray for me is priceless.

We are also blessed with two adult children who are believers in the Lord. Carey and Mark support us, encourage us, pray for us, and remind me at times of Wendy's needs. Carey knows intuitively how to take care of Wendy's health. She will tell me, "Dad, when you are out someplace and Mom says, 'I'm getting tired,' that is a signal to take her home *now*." Mark offers more subtly, "Maybe it is not such a good idea to plan that trip right now." How amazing to be able to learn from your children.

We have sometimes wasted time and energy trying to "see around the corner" and failed at predicting what the future holds. Several times Wendy has received diagnoses that carried the risk of death in the near future, and we braced for the worst only to find that it did not come. Many times we thought we were in for smooth sailing and ended up in an emergency room.

I would sometimes lie awake trying to calculate how much time we had left, wondering how to make the most of it, and frightfully imagining the prospect of living alone. I have since come to realize how right the Lord was in saying, "Sufficient unto the day are the troubles thereof." I now feel blessed by not knowing the timing of Wendy's or my death, since to know them would be to spend protracted days doing favorite things one last time, saying final goodbyes, and trying to make the best arrangements for the other one.

Instead, we accept that we do not know whether we will live another twenty years or another twenty minutes. So we try to see each day as both ordinary and a miracle— ordinary in the sense that we are not trying to cram in a lot of special events, and a miracle in the sense that we have been given something we cannot buy at any price—an additional day to live to God's glory.

Our marriage is a real blessing to us, and we realize that most people never have the closeness God has allowed us to share for forty-four years. We treasure what we have been given and are grateful for the prospect of a new life far better than this one.

I have shed tears and been through much agony in the past seventeen years, but God has used those tears to develop me into a better follower of Christ, a better husband, and a better father. I cannot know what is coming next. What I do know is that God will be in it with us.

Time Off

We should bestow the gift of time off to our caregivers as often as possible, and spouses especially need this. My husband and I have been best friends as well as spouses for forty-four years, and we do almost everything together outside of working hours. We have even written several books together, which is a real test of a friendship or marriage! Yet even with this close relationship Rick needs time to relax and forget about the illness that looms so large in our lives.

Before I was sick, most of Rick's hobbies involved spending time with me, so I encouraged him to take up golf. For Christmas I bought him a subscription to a golf magazine and gift certificates for the nearby golf range. I cannot play myself, but I sometimes go with him and drive the cart if he is golfing alone.

I encourage him to take lessons and to play regularly with his friends. He sometimes "complains" that I always want him to have fun. I see this as an investment in his peace, his future enjoyment, and our relationship. Nobody can be a caregiver all the time, and when he has time off from me, he returns to the task of loving a sick wife happier and with more energy.

Another critical component of this time off is interaction with other healthy adults. I realized early in my sickness that Rick had only a few close friends and that he did not spend much time with them. Carey noticed this also and encouraged her dad to grow closer to a few friends who could support him. One special friendship he formed during these years with a man also named Rick still thrives sixteen years later. The two Ricks now live three hours apart but talk often, sharing the ups and downs of their lives.

Every morning Rick takes our dog, Dante, for a long walk. For years his good friend Allen has walked with them every Tuesday, bringing his dog as well. Their friendship has grown stronger due to this time together; they depend on one another, share daily cares and larger concerns, and spur one another on to follow God's lead. Every other Wednesday Rick has lunch with Dom, another great friend.

I also encourage him to make phone calls to friends far and near. He often retires to his office for an hour or more, talking over important and trivial things with friends who care about him. I love to hear him laughing from the next room.

Not all caregivers can leave their loved ones for extended periods of time. Our friend, Joe, for instance, needs someone with him twenty-four hours a day. But his wife, Ethel, awakens several hours earlier than Joe in order to have daily time for herself. She has also arranged for a friend to come by one afternoon a week to so that she has time out of the house and can see friends for lunch or coffee. Thanks to the loving care of their children, she has even been able to go away overnight.

When we are willing to accept aid from others, we can usually find some relief from the constant drain of caregiving.

Time Together

Rick and I also need time alone, so we have always prioritized time away from home. When a couple lives with chronic illness, much of their communication centers on "pilot to co-pilot talk": who is picking up which child when, what the dinner plans are, which parent will attend which event when dates conflict. We need extended periods of time together without the distractions of home to talk about long-term goals, current fears, or enjoyable memories.

Often I am not really able to travel far from home. So we have learned to get away locally. During one especially cold and snowy winter, even for Michigan, many of our friends made trips to the warmth and sunshine of the South. Not able to do this, we booked the "snuggle special" at our local hotel: a suite with a Jacuzzi. We told our friends we were "going to Florida" for two days, got a sitter for the dog, drove the mile to the hotel, laughed when the clerk asked us if we wanted a map of the area, and sat in our Jacuzzi until we got too warm. We pretended the snow piled outside our window was white beach sand, watched movies on the large-screen television, and enjoyed the mammoth breakfast buffet. The next day we visited several local places we do not often get to, went out for a good dinner, and came home happily to the dog and the telephone messages. We had so much fun we are thinking of "going to Florida" again soon.

Spending even a few days away from people and household chores renews us. Think about ways to save regularly for such get-aways, perhaps putting money you might have spent for a fast-food meal in a jar and cooking your own hamburgers at home or taking a brown-bag lunch to work. Your weekend away will be well worth it.

Sometimes my body simply will not allow me to go away; then we take vacation days at home. We shut the curtains; ignore the phone and doorbell; spend as much time as we want talking together, reading, or playing music; and go out or order in meals. We even have "pajama days" when we don't get out of our bathrobes all day. Home vacations require advanced planning but will refresh your spirits.

Our Love Is What Is Important to Our Families

I continually face the challenge of feeling that I should be *doing* something for those I love. I naturally think of ways to help them, from small things like baking cookies to large things like cleaning someone's house for them. I must sort these impulses to avoid being physically exhausted.

One day when I wasn't feeling up to an actual walk, Rick and I took a "lying-down walk." After talking for a few minutes about his work, he suddenly said, "I really like you. I'm glad you're my friend." That day I had begun to feel quite useless because I hadn't finished anything on my to-do list. My immediate internal response to Rick's comment was "Why does he like me? I can't even do anything." But as he elaborated, I realized that he really just enjoys my friendship.

Rick, Carey, and Mark appreciate that I listen to them, care about them, pray for them, and support them. Fundamentally, they enjoy my perspective on life, my humor, my faith, and my personality. God has made us friends. I don't have to do anything except be their wife and mother to make them happy.

I have also learned that my family doesn't love me because of how I look. When I was young I had a thin body, but I now have a "prednisone belly." In spite of being in a normal weight range, steroids cause my stomach to bloat, and a digestive disorder exacerbates that problem. Long-term steroid use has also given me permanent chipmunk cheeks. Rashes come and go.

Sleep deprivation gives me dark circles under my eyes. I have many scars.

In short, I feel like I only resemble the woman Rick married all those years ago, while he still looks quite a bit like he did in his high school graduation photo. But Rick still looks at me with eyes of love that see past the scars. When you find this kind of love, protect and nourish it. Do not spend time worrying about being beautiful in the world's eyes.

Learning to Spend Our Days Wisely

My good friend Catherine has been battling cancer for almost three years. Some days are good, some not so good. Her faith sustains and encourages her through both. Catherine had always been the picture of health, and she struggles now, realizing that she has only a few hours' worth of energy every day. What should she do with it? She wants to walk with her husband, play with her son, talk with her daughter, and pursue her music and reading. But if she does these things with her hours, who will buy the groceries and make dinner? And perhaps even more important, how can she let her husband know how she *really* feels and when she needs help? How does she make it less confusing to her family that she may be "well" one minute and exhausted the next?

When you are sick, you constantly use part of your energy to heal and part just to get through mundane tasks that you used to do effortlessly. This, obviously, leaves less energy for the things you *want* to do. When I first became sick, this frustrated me. Ironically, I have even less energy now, but I am enjoying my waking hours more, due to two new strategies.

First, I have internalized the attitude of gratitude that I spoke about earlier. Every morning when I awaken, I thank God for another day on this earth doing whatever He would have me do. Having faced death many times, I understand how precious each day is and how carefully I should spend it.

I try to remember to ask God's grace for each hour during the day as well. Before my illnesses, I was a very productive person in the world's terms. I taught college, administered a department at my university, counseled patients in a private practice, published books and articles, homeschooled two terrific children, volunteered for various organizations, and worked at being a good wife. Fortunately God was about to teach me that these "accomplishments" were leading me away from Him and what He really wanted me to be producing.

My overly committed life did not allow for interruptions, and I was impatient with surprises that impacted my tight schedule. After all, when you are doing as much as I was doing, you must keep on schedule just to keep your head above water. Even good things such as a friend dropping by unexpectedly could annoy me.

I'm thankful that God taught me, "A man's pride brings him low, but a man of lowly spirit gains honor" (Proverbs 29:23). Since my physical health has slowed my pace, I have learned that interruptions often provide the most productive and wonderful moments in my day. When a neighbor stops by to talk just when I am sitting down to write, I immediately send up a prayer that I will be the friend she needs at that moment. When my son calls to invite himself to dinner on a night I was planning to pay the bills, I thank God for children who want to spend time with me. When a lonely and chatty elderly friend calls just as I am about to take a nap, I ask God to give me an understanding of her and patience in my responses. I can nap later. God always answers these prayers. I always gain from the encounters.

Second, I have learned to prioritize tasks, considering carefully the ones on which I want to spend my energy. My beloved grandfather once told me that the most important tasks of growing up were to learn how to spend our time and our money. Illness teaches me daily that we really do spend our time; nobody steals it from us. We should budget time just as we budget our money.

I now keep lists of activities separated into three priority levels. My level 1 list consists of things that I really do have to do, preferably today. These include continuing tasks such as exercise, prayer, Bible study, and making meals. Added to these are doctor's appointments, phone calls to check on test results, picking up medicines, and buying groceries. I complete these tasks with my first energy of the day because I cannot easily put them off.

My second list includes "keeping up" tasks that I would like to accomplish this week. These are things that help me maintain order in my life, such as throwing out old magazines or picking up the house so that Rick can vacuum. Some of them can be accomplished daily, but most pile up for me, and I address them occasionally.

The long-term tasks on the third list represent forward progress. Organizing the family photos or sewing a new set of curtains qualifies as a "forward progress" task. These tasks will remain done for a long time. I can plan to work on them and then feel good about having accomplished them. I incorporate some of these tasks into my week even if I must postpone some of the "keeping up" items to find the time. Most of us are energized by finishing something that we have wanted to do for a long time. I encourage you to let some dust lie while you finish a woodworking project, hang some family photos, or arrange flowers you dried years ago. Progress can satisfy the soul in a way that keeping up cannot.

As you make your three lists, commit to spending some time every day enjoying one of your passions. I love to play the piano. A good book will keep me happy for hours. I truly enjoy baking. Needlework fascinates me. I believe God created us with these passions and that He rejoices when we follow the passions He has given us.

Once you have set your priorities, consider what you can ask or pay someone else to do. Going to Wendy's one night a week or ordering in pizza every Friday removes the pressure of preparing a meal and allows for good conversation. Allowing friends to take your children for an afternoon frees up precious one-on-one time for a couple facing illness together. Perhaps you should consider spending vacation money that you can't use because of your illness to hire a twice-a-month housekeeper. Invest the energy and time you save in your family relationships.

Finally, share your lists with your family. Let them know that they will always be your highest earthly priority but that mundane tasks will occasionally exhaust your limited energy. Explain why you might choose to follow your passion for walking or feeding the birds before you help them with their homework or listen to them talk about their days. Describe how you feel when your energy evaporates unexpectedly and you simply cannot fulfill an expectation.

The truth is that illness changes your life forever. Your response to this truth will make the difference in how well your family does with your being sick. As you consider resources that will allow your family to thrive, learn to think outside the box. Do not reach the end of your days or the end of your ability to do what you want wondering why you did not fulfill your most important dreams.

Remembering What God Wants From Us

I learned one of life's most important lessons from my physical inability to do things for my family. Several years ago I was in a lupus flare that drained my energy and caused tremendous pain. My good friend Roz had been faithful in praying for me through this time. One day she called to share that this period of poor health could be a time for me to learn more about God and to rest in His love for me. Her words rang true.

Sickness opened space in my life to let God's love pour over me and sink into my heart.

Suddenly I realized that God does not care if I accomplish anything during my days; He cares about my relationship with Him. God wants me to be His friend, just as Rick and the children want me to be their friends. He wants me to learn about Him, listen to Him every day, and care about what He cares about. I am grateful that He has never given up on pursuing friendship with me and that He has revealed to me how small my idea of knowing Him has been. No matter what happens to my body, I can serve God every day.

In Summary

1. As much as possible, have a "full disclosure agreement" with your family, letting them know medical information when you know it.

2. Dare to have the difficult conversations with your loved ones about your death and other issues.

3. Happily give your caregivers time off.

4. Spend quality time with your family.

5. Use your time and energy carefully, keeping a joyful spirit and prioritizing tasks.

6. Realize that God wants your friendship, not your accomplishments.

Stand on Your Porch and Scream

Carey J. Wallace

They had just finished doing the dishes, and now they were planning her mother's funeral. The man at the funeral parlor had given her mother a list of funeral options and prices, which Jean was reading upside down as her mother talked.

"I don't want you to be worried because we're doing this now," her mother was saying. "I'm not in any more danger than I was before."

Seventy-five prayer cards cost twenty-five dollars, she read as her mother lied. The next operation had about a fifty-fifty chance of killing her. About half of the people who had done what her mother was about to do had died.

"So I wanted to see how you guys would want it to be. Because I won't be here," her mother said. "You're the important ones. I want you to be happy."

"Then don't die," Jean said. Driving the body to the church within twenty miles was a hundred and fifteen dollars, and then they got a quarter for every extra mile after that.

"I want to have a mushroom," her brother said, "when I die. I want to have a big marble mushroom for my gravestone, encased in a square glass box and with my name on it and some random date. Not the date I died. Like the first time I played my guitar or something."

"When did you first play your guitar?" Jean asked.

"I don't remember," he said.

"I don't want to be buried," she said. "I want to be cremated and have my ashes put out at the lake or scattered in a field of daisies or something. I wouldn't like to be underground. I don't want part of me to be left here. I don't want anyone to see me if I'm dead."

"It's not like it's embarrassing," her brother said. "It's not like people are allowed to make fun of you when you're dead."

"I just don't want to be in a box," she said. "I don't want to be underground."

Her father hadn't said anything at all yet, but he had moved his water glass three times.

"I wanted," said their mother, "to set this up without bothering you all. When I first went to the funeral home, I went in because I wanted a very simple burial within twenty-four hours. I wanted to have that on record so that you wouldn't have to deal with it if I was to die."

"Then why are we talking about this?" Mark asked.

"Well, the man thinks that a simple burial might not be the best way."

"That's his job," Jean said.

"The man I talked to was Don Cole," her mother said. "And he was very nice."

"He's paid," Mark said. Jean looked at him.

"He was very nice," their mother repeated. "And he, in fact, told me that if we are ever in a situation where we cannot pay for anything, that he would do my funeral for free."

Everyone was quiet.

Jean was furious. It wasn't fair that a person like her mother could die. It wasn't fair that a person who someone would do a funeral for free for would die.

"That's nice," Mark said, very quietly.

"What he told me that I hadn't thought of," their mother began again, "was that a lot of people can't get here in twenty-four hours. So a lot of people wouldn't have a chance to say good-bye. And even fewer would be able to come to a viewing,"

"A viewing?" Jean said. "I thought that you were going to have a simple burial."

"Yes," said her mother. "But there are other people besides you who will want to say good-bye."

"So?" Jean said. "I don't care."

"Well, it's for them, too," her mother said.

"Their mother didn't die," Jean said.

"I don't know," Mark said. "I don't know what would happen to me if you died. I'm scared I'd start spending all my time in my room in the dark listening to music with whiny guitar solos all the time."

Jean was quiet. She had thought about her mother dying only once before, and her main worry had been that she be alive until the winter formal so that she could sew a dress. Jean had learned from her mother how to sew shorts and blouses, but she still couldn't do anything with velvet. She didn't want to see her father cry, either.

She would be the one to take care of everything, she thought. Her father had gone to the airport after the first heart attack with one pair of jeans, wingtips, and no deodorant. Her brother had brought three boxes of tapes and a Walkman with no batteries and had left his travel case with all of his toothpaste and soap on the shelf next to the stereo.

She had sat in the Chinese restaurant where they went after seeing her mother in the hospital and written out lists of things they needed on the back of a napkin with her father's pen. Toothpaste. Soap. Tylenol. Donuts (for brkfst). Batteries. She had never made lists before.

"You're turning into Mom," Mark had said.

She had said, "No, I'm not," and put the Crest back because it was twenty-nine cents more expensive than Colgate.

Cremation cost the same as a simple burial in a very basic pine coffin.

"So there's no real price advantage in being cremated," her mother said. "It seems like I might as well just have a regular burial."

"Save God time and energy at the last judgment," Mark said. "Won't have to make you a whole new body."

"Then we have to decide if we want a viewing and a memorial service or not," her father said.

"I don't want to go to a viewing," Jean said.

"The viewing is very important, honey," her mother said.

"I don't want to go," Jean said. "When Sara's brother killed himself last summer, no one else in her family would go, and she stood there for a whole day with him there in the room dead."

"You don't have to stay all day," her mother said.

"I think that you need to see the body," her father said.

"Why?" Jean said. "So that I know she's really truly dead? I'll be there if she dies. I can see her in the hospital or whatever. She'll look more dead there than dressed up and wearing lipstick at the funeral parlor."

"Saying good-bye to the body can help you accept the fact of death," her mother said.

"I'm not stupid, Mom," Jean said. "Death is a pretty basic concept. I'm in the top of my class. I got an A in biology."

"Doesn't having a viewing mean you have to be embalmed?" Mark asked.

"I don't know," their mother said, picking up the price list. "I'm not sure if I want to be embalmed."

"I don't want to be embalmed," Jean said. "It's horrible."

"What's wrong with embalming?" her father asked. "All they do is insert two tubes. They take the blood out and put chemicals in. It's very simple."

"Embalming? Dad, are you kidding? They take your brains out through your nose. I just had this in class."

"They do not take your brains out through your nose," her father said, moving his water glass again and leaning back.

"They do, too," she said. "They have to take out everything or your organs start to smell. And they can't just crack your head open."

"The man did talk about it as a surgery," her mother said. "He said it was a surgery."

"It's like surgery," Jean said. "They take your brains out through your nose and fill you up with formaldehyde."

"I thought that was mummification," Mark said.

"It's mummification, too," Jean said.

"She's going to be buried," her father said.

"Well, who says you have to be buried anyway?" Jean said. "There are lots of other ways to get rid of a body. I mean, we're getting pretty ethnocentric.

"In Africa they do all sorts of other things. Sometimes they put people in jars and drain off the fluids over a period of months. And then they bury the bones and dig them up again in a few years to see if you're a good person or not."

"We just did aborigines in history," Mark said. "I know how to shrink heads now."

"And the spouse has to sit next to the jar and offer it food and cry every hour. Glad you don't live in Africa, Dad?"

Her father stared across the table just over her head. He looked sick. She looked away.

"In some cultures, the whole town has to go outside and scream once a day when someone dies. Do you think we could get people here to do that?"

"It's really easy to shrink a head, actually," Mark said.

"What if we put an ad in *The Chelsea Standard*?" Jean asked. "Instead of sending flowers, please stand on your porch at 2:30 and scream."

"Wanna hear how to do it?" Mark asked.

"No," their father said.

Their mother was quiet, but didn't look upset. Jean was on the edge of a laugh. She and Mark had done this on the day of their mother's original heart attack.

"What's up?" a friend had asked them as they were coming out of McDonald's.

"Not much," Mark had said.

"Doing anything tonight?"

"We're flying to St. Louis," Jean said. "My mother had a heart attack last night while she was away on business and is in an intensive care unit in Washington, Missouri. I was very mean to her on the phone when she called this morning because she woke me up." She had burst into giggles. She never giggled.

"We're actually leaving right now to catch the plane," Mark said, smiling. "Excuse us."

No one could ever tell if they were serious or not anyway, and their friend had just nodded. "There's a party at Scott's tonight if things fall through," he said as they left.

"We'll have to see how the nitroglycerin works," Mark called back. "Don't count on us."

"They're going to think we're horrible if you make us go to the visitation," Jean said.

"We'd just end up doing stand-up funeral comedy," Mark said.

Their mother looked at them.

"No," said Jean. "No. Mark would stand there and not say anything, and I'd be the one who consoled everyone because my mother died and their lives are going to be so bleak without you to dump all their problems on."

"Yeah," said Mark.

"And we'd have to pretend that they were making us feel better so that they could go home feeling useful. I don't want to do that," Jean said. "I don't want to be half sad. I don't want to have to smile and let a little tear run down when they say how wonderful you were, but not be able to scream at them for being worthless and alive when you're dead. I either want to go right back to life without a break or be able to leave and sit in some cabin somewhere by myself for a month and cry."

"I don't want to have to take care of other people," Jean said. "If we have a viewing I'd have to take care of other people."

"Let's have a viewing and Jean can stay home and watch TV," Mark said.

"Really," Jean said. "I can say good-bye before anyone else gets there and go home."

"I think that it's important that you see the body," her father said.

"Dad, I will. I just don't want to see other people."

"I think that would be alright, honey," her mother said.

"The Mom Psychological Damage stamp of approval," said Mark.

"Alright," said her father. "Have we made any decisions here?"

"I think this basic funeral package is the best thing," her mother said. "I'll just go ahead and be embalmed, and we can have viewing and a memorial service as simple as possible."

"Are we done?" Mark asked.

"No," their father said. He moved his water glass onto his napkin.

"What about flowers?" her mother asked. "I think I'm going to ask that the money go to charity instead."

"No flowers," Jean said. "Nana says she can't look at a lily without thinking about death. That would make me sick. I don't want there to be flowers."

"Are we going to give out any little things with the programs for them to remember the service by?" Mark asked. "Dead roses or something? Like funeral favors?"

"No, Mark," their father said.

Their mother smiled. "Little prayer cards," she said.

"Black noisemakers," said Jean.

They were all laughing, except their father.

"Can we try to bring this to a close?" he asked.

"Yes," said their mother. "I think I'll just tell Don that this is what we want. It should be a very nice service."

"I could live without going to it," Jean said.

"So could I," her mother said. She folded the price list and put it back in the envelope. "Did we have dessert?" she asked.

"No," their father said.

"There's peach frozen yogurt in the freezer downstairs," said Jean.

"Mark, why don't you run down and get it?" said their mother. She stood up and put the funeral papers in the kitchen cupboard in between the folders with the bills and the one for old report cards.

"That wasn't so bad," she said.

Jean smiled at her.

"No," their father said, and took a drink of water.

Chapter Four

~

Our Being Sick Affects Our Friends

<u>*You will learn:*</u>

- to easily communicate information to your friends
- to understand that others will not always understand
- to receive help
- to be a good friend

For the joy of human love,
Brother, sister, parent, child,
Friends on earth and friends above,
For all gentle thoughts, and mild,
Lord of all, to Thee we raise,
This our hymn of grateful praise.

FOLLIOTT PIERPONT

~

For over a decade, we have hosted a small-group Bible study at our house. One of the women, whose name, like mine, is Wendy, hates being the center of attention. If you were at a party and didn't know her, you might never notice her, and she would be happy with that. But Wendy has a keen mind and a loving heart and has become my special friend.

Years ago, when I had been in an automobile accident, Rick was out of town. He called Wendy, and she knocked on my door minutes after I arrived home and was wise enough just to hug me and let me cry until I calmed down.

Several years ago I was going through a particularly rough time physically. Wendy wrote me a letter expressing her feelings for me and letting me know she was praying for me. I know that her natural reticence made this difficult for her to do in person; I am certain it was not easy for her to do even in writing. I treasure the letter still.

One summer Wendy delivered a dozen jars of canned peaches to me because she knew I loved them and couldn't can them myself. Once I came home from a morning of doctors' appointments to discover that Wendy had weeded my entire garden while I was gone. She had checked the calendar hanging on my bulletin board so she knew when I would be out of the house. When I was healing from a surgery and an allergic reaction, she started arriving periodically with canned apricots or loaves of homemade bread. Recently, her husband, Allen, shared that she had trouble sleeping one night because she was worried about some of my health issues.

Wendy is my true sister in the Lord and cares for me as much as a biological sister ever could. She thinks about my needs and fills them with her talents as she is led. She never waits for me to ask her for help, but I know she is always standing by. Wendy shows God's love to me in concrete and spiritual ways, and I am very grateful to God for her friendship. I also feel sad that my being sick brings her pain.

Most of us have social relationships that are as important to us as our family relationships. We belong to churches, Bible studies, book groups, volunteer groups, clubs based on our hobbies and interests, and many other composites. We have friends from work, college, and from the area where we live. If we are so blessed, we have friends we've known since we were children. Because they all care about us, our illnesses affect them. Friends bring blessings. But taking care of your friends while you are sick can deplete the energy you and your family need to manage your illness.

Dealing with "the Public"

In times of medical crisis, your friends will want to keep in touch with you. But just furnishing them with current information can be exhausting. Phone calls take time and emotional energy. Re-telling the story of a painful medical experience many times, for instance, can wear down the strongest person. Your family's precious time should be spent instead on caring for you and being together.

Preserve your time and energy by providing information in ways that require less time and emotional energy. Use your e-mail system to keep your friends in the loop so that they don't overwhelm your family with many phone calls. Ask your friends for their e-mail addresses, create an address book for them, and assign the task of updating them to a friend or family member who is good at that sort of thing.

Blogs provide an even easier way to keep contact with others. Starting a blog and posting information on it periodically does not even require an e-mail list. People can access the blog any time without your contacting them. Find someone with blogging experience to start a blog for you if you are not familiar with this technology. If having your own blog seems daunting, social network services such as Facebook and MySpace offer simple ways to keep in contact.

Some of the larger hospital systems provide a free informational Internet service through their own servers. In fact, if you have been hospitalized for illness or injury or know of someone who has, you may have used CarePages.com, one of the most popular of these services. These resources enable families or friends to create a personalized Web site for patients. Friends and relatives who subscribe to the free service can read the latest news and information posted by the patient representative, view photos, and send messages to the patient and even receive e-mail notification whenever the patient representative posts an update. This can be a godsend that allows friends to get updates without burdening you or your family. If your hospital offers this service, ask one good friend or family member to be your public relations person and manage your Web site.

When you are in public—at church, for instance—where people know some but not all of your circumstances, answer their questions honestly, but don't dwell on the details with everyone. Most people don't know how to respond to bad news. Rather than burdening questioners with an awkward moment, provide information and move on. My friend Catherine has found it useful to respond to such questions truthfully and briefly and then to ask, "And how are *you*?" Catherine's listening and responding to them changes the subject effectively and politely.

In reality, there are only a few people who really want to know how you are doing. Many of them are politely concerned but not committed to knowing or caring for you and your family. A few are good friends. You may want to have your spouse call them to personally convey word of a hospitalization or surgical outcome. I have given Rick a card that lists key people (and their phone numbers) to call for prayers and updates. It helps him communicate more efficiently and not forget anyone who should be called.

What Being a Good Friend Looks Like

Proverbs tells us "a friend loves at all times, and a brother is born for adversity" (Proverbs 17:17). But how does this play out in real life? I have faced a myriad of medical problems, but usually God has graciously given me one thing on my plate at a time. One autumn the crises seemed to come so quickly I could not even research one new diagnosis and form a plan of action with my doctors before the next diagnosis came. I was exhausted and sick.

One morning I received a phone call telling me that a CT scan that I knew had revealed bladder cancer had also uncovered another problem: sclerotic mesenteritis. This incurable rare disease had been creating havoc in my digestive system for some time. Now I was not only feeling sick but also sorry for myself and discouraged. I knew that this mood would pass, but at that moment I decided that I would not talk about the diagnosis with anyone until it did pass.

The phone rang. My friend Diane was in town and wondered if she could stop by for a few minutes. Normally I am delighted to see Diane. She brings the grace and light of Jesus wherever she goes and has faithfully walked with me for years. This day I hesitated, but agreed to the visit. After all, I reasoned, just because she was here did not mean I had to share my feelings with her.

Knowing some of the new physical challenges I had been facing, Diane asked if this was a discouraging time for me. I immediately began to sob and spent the next hour talking openly with her about my situation. Most of the other people in my life had been either too oblivious or too affected by the situation to be able to talk about it. I had done what I usually do—tried to help them to be more comfortable—rather than sharing myself with them.

In contrast, Diane recognized by my tone of voice on the phone that something was not right and waded right in to stand by me. What a blessing she gave me: the freedom to talk openly about my new health concerns! Once again she offered me the gift of good friendship.

God has graciously used my illness to teach me to receive love from family and friends as well as how to be a good friend. I offer what I have learned not only for those who cope with illness, but for their caregivers as well.

Listening and Responding Well

How can we be good friends and teach others to be the same? First, practice listening. James 1:19 counsels us to "be quick to listen [and] slow to speak." How often we do the opposite: when faced with a problem, we naturally want to offer a solution. But we should not jump in with a solution before a friend has had the chance to explain a problem entirely.

People usually just need to talk things through with someone to come to a better understanding of their own issues. Our friends can only explore their rational and irrational feelings and fears with us when we are really open to hearing them. They almost *never* want us to fix something, but rather to understand them.

The next time someone honors you by sharing his or her personal thoughts and feelings, close your mouth and open your ears. Don't take a pause in the conversation as a green light for your advice. Instead, encourage your friend to continue by saying things like, "How did that feel?" "I can't imagine how you must have felt." "I am so sorry that you had to go through that." "That must be really difficult." Share only comments that will help your friend continue to talk.

People often say things to me like, "You look good. You must be feeling good." When I am spruced up for a family occasion, one of the kids might even say this as a joke because we have heard it so many times from others. I finally understand that these friends are often really saying, "I don't know how to deal with the fact that you are chronically ill. I want you to be better, so sometimes I pretend that you are." Alternatively people may try to encourage me, not understanding the nature of chronic illness. A good friend will avoid making these comments. To be a good friend, ask the kinds of questions I just suggested. As a person with an illness, forgive such comments from others, understanding that these friends truly don't realize what they are saying and how it makes you feel.

People may also inadvertently hurt our feelings or create awkwardness by offering suggestions about the ways we should handle illness. Friends and acquaintances have offered me information about potential elixirs of health, diets, and mind-sets that are guaranteed to cure everything. They mean well, and I have learned to thank them kindly while telling them we are satisfied with the treatments we are currently using.

Human beings do not like to concede that they are not in charge of the universe and their destinies. We hate being unable to stop the pain of a loved one. So we sometimes pretend that there is something that can be done when all avenues really have already been explored. If you learn of a new treatment possibility, by all means share the information. But remember that good friends are willing to simply live in an ill person's reality without trying to make him or her better.

Also, good friends should endeavor to understand the world from the other's perspective, whatever his or her circumstances. My friend Szonja wrote me once "I hope that you are doing well by your special and personal definition." The more people I know intimately, the more I realize that most of us go through life showing the world only the tip of our iceberg. We hide the most painful, embarrassing, fearsome aspects of our lives. If we are fortunate and patient, a few friends will let us into their hidden places, and we will come to understand why they act and react to things as they do.

Most of us, however, will never know deeply personal matters about the people we interact with, even those we count as friends. Because of this, we must consciously dispense grace in large measure every day. We are ignorant, in the true sense of the word, of the load others are carrying. We often do not know their background. We can never understand fully what they believe. But we can love them unswervingly, regardless of how they treat us at any given moment. A good friend offers grace without conditions.

Praying

One of the blessings of friendship is being able to pray with and for a friend. Sometimes our prayers will be a direct response to a request. My friends have asked for prayers for everything from renewed health to a greater closeness with the Lord. I have asked people just to pray for me when I did not have words to describe my condition. Charles Stanley suggests using Colossians 1:9–12 as a basis for prayer when you don't know the specific needs of your friend. I keep a copy of this passage on my dresser and pray through it for several people every morning and evening.

> *Since the day we heard about you, we have not stopped praying for you and asking God to fill you with the knowledge of his will through all spiritual wisdom and understanding. And we pray this in order that you may live a life worthy of the Lord and may please him in every way: bearing fruit in every good work, growing in the knowledge of God, being strengthened with all power according to his glorious might so that you may have great endurance and patience, and joyfully giving thanks to the Father, who has qualified you to share in the inheritance of the saints in the kingdom of light.*

Other times God will direct our prayers to His purpose for our friends. I have often prayed for a person for no special reason only to discover later that he or she needed prayer at that particular moment. Often when I hear distress in a friend's voice on the other end of the phone line, I pray immediately that God will direct my conversation with him or her. God always answers these prayers.

I strongly believe that as we remain open, God will tell us how to lift others up to Him. God connects people through himself. In order to be available for this process, we must stay in constant contact with Him through prayer.

Doing without Being Asked

A good friend rarely waits to be asked to help. Because of the ongoing relationship and prodding from the Lord, a friend often senses a need and acts on it before the person in need can articulate the problem. After my third heart attack, Rick called my oldest friend, Maggie, whom I have known since we were both thirteen years old. Maggie lived about eight hours away and had a full-time job teaching at a university. But her love for me was put into action immediately upon hearing from Rick.

Within the day, Maggie walked into my hospital room, one of the most touching moments of my life. She did not cure me. She did not clean my house, confer with my doctors, eliminate the sadness and fear from my family's eyes, or make the hospital food good to eat. She simply loved me and showed this by being with me at a time when I needed her love. Maggie sat by my bed and talked, listened, or rested, depending on my signals at the moment. She rolled my IV pole when I moved from one room to another and made sure nothing was left behind. I will never forget those hours we spent together, and I cannot write about them even today, sixteen years later, without tears in my eyes. I did not have to ask her for anything; she simply ministered to me as she saw my needs.

Accepting Reality

Even your close friends and family members sometimes have trouble accepting the reality of a chronic illness or a terminal prognosis. I remember going to visit my mother and father just after I found out I had lupus. I had been sick and unable to visit them for several weeks. When I walked in the door, Mom hugged me and asked what the doctors had told us.

"I have lupus," I said.

"No, you don't," my dad responded.

Dad's response was not scientific but emotional. He loved me and did not want me to have lupus, a disease that had claimed the life of a childhood friend of mine many years earlier. Therefore, in his mind, I did not have lupus. I absolutely understood his reaction, and I may well have responded exactly the same way if one of my children brought me that news. Parents hate to stand by while one of their children suffers, helpless to offer relief. Dad was always the provider in our family, the one you could depend on. He could not fix the lupus, and his first reaction was to deny it.

Over time Dad and Mom both accepted the lupus diagnosis and my many other health challenges with grace and love. They came to visit me in the hospital, cared for the kids, made meals, made homemade applesauce with apples from their orchard, called when they couldn't visit, and let me know how much they loved me even when I was just lying there waiting out a heart attack with the nitro drip. We gave each other time and space to accept the situation, and the investment paid dividends.

I have learned not to be angry at people's inability to handle my reality. Once I was scheduled for a necessary surgery during which I had a twenty-percent chance of dying, a frightening prospect for me and my family. When my husband shared this with an acquaintance at church, the response he received was a chipper, "Well, that's an eighty-percent chance that she will live through it!" Obviously this person could not walk in our shoes and understand. A simple "I am so sorry" would have been useful and confirming, but he was unable to say that.

Because accepting reality is a process, we must learn to be patient with our friends and family. We like to think that they will immediately be able to understand our situations. But empathy is learned, and many of us have not had good models of empathy in our lives. Forgiving those who do not have this ability saves energy for healing. Perhaps they can learn from you in the future when you honor them with an empathetic response as a good friend. At the least, forgiving them and moving on can be integral to your own acceptance of the reality of life with illness.

Putting Trust in Friends

We all need a few friends with whom we can be honest and completely forthcoming. These people really *do* want to know how you are. They remember which doctors you are going to visit and which tests you had last week and want to know the results so that they can pray for you or help you in other ways. With these people, you can be sad, glad, or mad. You should be truthful with them; do not pretend that you are strong all the time, and do let them help you.

Diane has hung in with me for so long that I've allowed her to know me on the inside. She knows I am not just a strong, courageous survivor who counsels other people, but a person who sometimes gets angry, frightened, and discouraged. I call her to ask her to pray for me, and she calls me when she needs prayer. When Diane comes to visit, she doesn't care what I wear or whether my house is clean or dirty; we just enjoy time together. She thinks about my needs. When I was confined to my house for an extended time, she invested hours creating a painting for me to hang where I could look at it any time. She is truly a blessing from God.

Raised in a family that emphasized self-reliance, I had to learn to trust friends like Diane, Wendy, and many others to know me and love me. I encourage you to be careful not to complain all the time but to let key friends participate in your inner life. Likewise, listen to your friends' problems and concerns, even when you are not feeling well yourself. You will undoubtedly feel better after helping someone you love by listening. Mutually supportive friendship is a rare gift from God and should be both exercised and treasured.

It Is Blessed to Receive

God has given me the gift of understanding and aiding people. Most of my life I spent my energy helping others. However, I am embarrassed to say, I sometimes prided myself on helping others. This made it difficult for me to accept help, even when I obviously needed it.

I'm thankful that my friend Roz pointed out to me that my pride deprived my family of aid they needed and my friends of the blessing of helping a loved one. Roz's good counsel led me to accept help with things that needed to be done such as housework, grocery shopping, and transportation to doctors' appointments. Later I learned to enjoy help with nonessentials like cooking meals so that my family could spend some of our time together not doing chores.

Recently Mark and Rick were rebuilding the front porch on Mark's century-old house. Rick cut his hand badly with a handsaw and drove himself to the emergency room for stitches while Mark struggled to finish the project by himself before dark since the tenants in the house had no other way to enter their apartment. I called our friend Allen, who came to Mark's rescue. He left his family, drove half an hour, and spent another two hours finishing the project with Mark. When we thanked him for his generosity, he answered, "That's what family is for."

We are blessed to have friends who have become family, in the sense that we are all God's children, and also because we love one another with everlasting, forgiving, caring love. We can appreciate these brothers and sisters especially if we haven't been blessed with this kind of love in our biological family. I have actually learned to believe my friends when they say that taking me to an appointment is one of the highlights of their week or that they are really glad to go to the pharmacy for me.

God's Friendship

Like all of us, my friend Wendy sometimes lies awake at night worrying about things she knows she has no control over. When she shared this one night at Bible study, the entire group could relate. We all have times when we wish we could talk with someone in the wee hours of the morning. Wendy imagined a solution that struck a chord with the entire group. We could install green lights on our phones: if we were awake in the middle of the night, we would turn them on and our friends would know they could call us.

Obviously our phones have no such light even in today's technologically advanced world. But God's green light is always on. We never receive an answering machine message from Him saying He will call back when it is convenient. He models the best kind of friendship.

In a recent Bible study we were challenged to spend a week letting God ask *us* questions rather than our questioning God. Despite my years of discipleship and study, I found God asking me things like, "Why don't you really trust me with your children's lives?" and "What exactly is it about the future of your body's problems that you think I can't handle?" God is not our "buddy in the sky." But He does know, understand, and care more than any earthly friend could. He is, after all, God, and we are commanded and encouraged to trust in Him and be still before Him. If we remember nothing else about friendship, we must remember this.

I urge you to nurture your earthly and heavenly friendships now, while God gives you the opportunity. Spend the time to invest in friendship. Remember that only two things really matter on this earth: our relationship to God and our relationship to others. Cleaning the house is way down on the list of important activities. Sitting over a cup of hot cocoa with someone you love is very high. It is that simple.

In Summary

1. Find ways to get medical information to your friends that do not sap you and your family of energy.

2. Forgive the public for not understanding everything you are going through.

3. Nurture a few good friendships now.

4. Give your friends the gift of being able to help you.

5. Nurture your relationship with God and others.

Chapter Five

Relying on God

You will learn:

- to focus on God
- to understand why God is trustworthy
- to rely on God rather than yourself
- to respond to God according to His wishes

We have no power to face this vast army
that is attacking us. We do not know what to do,
but our eyes are upon you.

2 CHRONICLES 20:12

I had interviewed for my dream job teaching at a private high school and was hoping to hear the school's decision when Rick and I left for a long-awaited vacation. We asked our friend Tracy to check our mail every day for a letter from the school and to call us if it arrived. When we returned, I realized the letter had arrived, but Tracy hadn't recognized the small envelope it had come in, although the return address was clearly the school's. I called immediately, but the principal had given the job to someone else, thinking I was not interested.

At first I was so furious with Tracy that I could not even talk to her. I believed that the teaching job was perfect for me. My other work prospects paled in comparison. Nothing could console me for the loss. Tracy felt terrible, of course, but I did not forgive her. Eventually I calmed down, and we resumed the relationship. I am still ashamed of my behavior at the time.

We can all think of a time when someone we trusted let us down. I spent almost a year after that in various dead-end temporary positions. I even tried to sell life insurance, for me a sure sign of desperation, since I have no ability in this area. But because I did not have a teaching position, I was able to think about pursuing other careers. During this time outside the classroom, I realized that what I had enjoyed the most about teaching was the interaction with my students. I liked counseling them, helping them evaluate their lives, and guiding them to choose new behaviors. My work as the speech and drama coach opened opportunities for one-on-one discussion with my students, many of whom shared eagerly with me.

However, I would often come to a point where I did not know what to do or say. I realized that I needed additional training to become more useful to my students. So I enrolled in graduate school in the clinical social work program at the University of Connecticut, majoring in marriage and family counseling. When I completed my master's degree in social work (MSW), I began private practice in counseling, working with people of all ages but specializing in teenagers and their families. I loved the work, and God blessed the results. I counseled, taught college courses, wrote books, and raised my children on a flexible schedule. If I had continued to work as a high school teacher, I would have had great difficulty accomplishing these things.

I understand in hindsight what God knew at the time: being hired for my "dream job" would have delayed my training for a career that better used my talents. God used Tracy's mistake to help me find my spot in His kingdom and gave me the fallow period after that to focus on my next steps. Today I praise Him for his kindness in *not* giving me what I wanted.

From Self-Reliance to God-Reliance

Probably the most important lesson I have learned from my illness is to rely on God and not on myself. I had always been a bright, self-motivated, energetic person. I made plans and carried them out. Although I gave lip service to God being the center of the universe, I routinely ignored this fact and tried to control the world around me. In fact, even now if I have an extended period of time when I feel healthy, I often jump right back into this "self-directed" way of acting. I make lists and assume I will be able to accomplish *my* goals without worrying much about whether or not they are *God's* goals. When we do things by ourselves, we do not allow God the opportunity to do things with and through us.

A friend once told me that the last time he prayed was during a high school chemistry test. Many contemporary Americans could echo this confession. Illness often breaks people out of this cycle. When we enjoy health, we feel self-reliant. When illness enters our lives, we realize how dependent we are on things we cannot control.

People often ask others to pray for a loved one who is sick. We frequently hear "there's nothing more to do except pray," as if prayer functions only as a last resort. In these situations we finally understand that the God of the universe is almighty; we are not. When faced with catastrophic illness we must acknowledge this fact, perhaps for the first time.

Focusing on God

God wants us to bring all of our problems to Him through prayer, and He receives them as we are able to bring them. However, I believe that we are most helped through prayer when we open our entire lives to Him during all the moments of all our days. He does not want us to toss up our difficulties first thing in the morning and then be so busy during the day that we don't hear His answers. Especially when we are coping with a chronic problem such as illness, God can best help us when we pray as Jehoshaphat did. Faced with overwhelming odds against the Moabites, Ammonites, and Meunites he prayed, "We do not know what to do, but our eyes are on you" (2 Chronicles 20:12).

My Great Aunt Edith had a favorite saying: "Glance at your problems; gaze at Jesus." I believe that in one way or another, Jesus is God's solution to every problem we have; we just don't always understand or accept that.

Why We Find It Difficult to Trust God

We have never seen God, so our tendency is to ascribe human characteristics to His personality. This makes sense, because from childhood our parents, family friends, and public figures function as our yardsticks for behavior. When we are young we think that they are God-like. As we grow, however, we discover that human beings are fallible, selfish, time-limited, weak, and prideful. In contrast, God is omniscient, all loving, omnipresent, all-powerful, and gracious.

God Transcends Time

For instance, *while we think in the short-term, God thinks over all time*. Our health problems loom large on our horizons. Crippling arthritis, pending surgery, cancer—all of these challenges dominate our thoughts day and night if we allow them to. God, however, knows that our lives on earth are short compared to our lives in eternity and that days when we struggle with physical illness are fleeting. Theories abound as to why God allows suffering on earth. What we do know is that our suffering helps us learn to trust in God. This is our major task while here on earth, and Hebrews 11 describes the nature and power of this trust by examining the lives of well-known Old Testament believers: The writer of Hebrews tell us that Moses "persevered because he saw him who is invisible" (v. 27); after describing the circumstances of various Old Testament believers, he summarizes, "These were all commended for their faith, yet none of them received what had been promised. God had planned something better for us so that only together with us would they be made perfect" (vv. 39–40).

God Is Omniscient

Another reason for our difficulty in trusting God's plan is that *earth is limited in scope and heaven is not*. We believe in time schedules, deadlines, and being able to find everything on the Internet. God sees things on a continuum and understands all things because He created all things. He sees, at once, our past, present, and future. He knows what is best for us because of this perspective. As a result of our limited knowledge, we focus on our immediate problems and our desire to solve them. God, instead, focuses on our development and our relationship with Him and other people in our lives.

My friend Sue had been recently diagnosed with rheumatoid arthritis when we spoke after a church service. Tears welled up in her eyes because of her pain and the diagnosis. But she told me unequivocally, "Life is good because I am learning to rely upon God in ways I never have." Relying on God is so important that He is willing to allow us to experience pain in order to learn it.

A few days after our daughter Carey was born, a nurse came into the room to take blood from her ankle. Carey screamed loudly, and I was as tortured as she was. I asked the nurse if this test was absolutely necessary. She explained that it would show the presence or absence of a fatal disease that could be treated if found early. In my own strength I would probably have decided that to love my child, I should not subject her to such pain. But I covered my ears and allowed the nurse to proceed. If my love for Carey had been limited to ending her short-term suffering, I might have stopped the test and exposed Carey to dangerous future consequences.

Parents understand that we must sometimes allow our children to experience pain to keep them healthy in the future. Our children often do not understand, and their questioning eyes may accuse us of not caring that they are being hurt. We bear the anger and confusion because we can see farther than they can and have more information than they have. We know what they need, and we supply it.

This is also true of our relationship with God. His Word tells us, "The Lord is my shepherd, I shall not be in want" (Psalm 23:1). Since His Word is true, this means that when we *believe* we need something we are not receiving, we do not *actually* need it. In fact, what we desire may not be good for us. God's love provides all that we need even when we do not understand His methods.

God's Timing Is Perfect

God also provides what we need at the exact moment we need it. I love the story Corrie ten Boom tells in *The Hiding Place* about when she was a small child going on a train trip with her father. She wants to hold her ticket herself, but her father tells her she must wait until they get onto the train. He explains to her that he will give her the ticket at the exact moment she needs it, not sooner and not later, just as God gives us what we need to cope with life's trials when we need it. Corrie clings to this lesson through years of horror in German concentration camps and grows closer to God as she waits.

Recently Dr. Leonard, the physical medicine and rehabilitation doctor who has kept me mobile for many years, prescribed physical therapy for a chronic disc problem in my back, exacerbated by my falling on the concrete floor of our garage. I had previously received physical therapy at the University of Michigan Hospital, but I am not able to drive that far by myself anymore and hesitated to pressure my friends and family to take me back and forth several times a week. Instead I called the local hospital clinic for its first available appointment, almost a month away. I unhappily resigned myself to the long wait.

A few days later I saw my massage therapist and told her about my long wait for an appointment. She told me about Marcy Boughton, a new physical therapist in town who had produced marvelous results in several patients they shared. I made a much earlier appointment with Marcy, who proved to be the best physical therapist I have ever worked with as well as a friend. In fact, she has made so much progress with my body that I can often drive myself the short distance to see her.

My finding Marcy at exactly the right moment was not coincidence but God's timing. Years ago I would have asked my doctor to insist on an earlier appointment at the hospital physical therapy clinic and missed this wonderful thing God had planned for me. God has graciously taught me to let Him handle the timing of things in my life. When I manage to do this, He brings me where I need to be.

God Is Love

Unlike humans, God always does the loving thing. My mother used to tell a story about her Grandma Tozer, whose strong faith in God had guided her through many trials. One day Grandma, who lived with my mom's family, had made a double batch of her famous sour cream cookies and then went out to run errands. When she returned she found Mom and her friends sitting on the living room floor, just finishing the last of the cookies. Grandma gasped, took a deep breath, and said, "Well, I guess I'd better make another batch." Guided by the love of her Master, Grandma Tozer gifted my mother with love rather than hurting her with wrath or even disapproval.

We are naturally selfish and often make decisions based on that selfishness. God, in contrast, always acts in accordance with His loving nature. Whether we are aware of it or not, He always sends us "showers of blessings" (Ezekiel 34:26), including physical comforts, emotional and spiritual encouragement, peace, and security. Often He allows challenges that help us to grow in our relationship with Him, the biggest blessing of all.

In sharp contrast to ours, God's priorities are always correct, and He does not withhold love as we so often do. John reminds us "From the fullness of his grace we have all received one blessing after another" (John 1:16). Surely I should be passing this blessing on to those He puts in my path daily. When I adopt this perspective, perhaps rather than being annoyed at challenges, I can adopt Grandma Tozer's stance and thank God that we have the ingredients to make another batch of cookies.

God's Solutions Are Peaceful

God's ways always bring contentment, and our ways often bring discontent. When I lost my "dream job," I allowed the incident to knock my entire life off balance for weeks. Nothing would please me. I was unreasonably unhappy in the dead-end work I was doing.

If I had simply acknowledged that God was in control of my life and looked for His lesson in the situation, I would have moved more quickly out of my grief to a place of contentment. Instead of asking, "Why did this happen?" I should have been asking, "What do you want to teach me now, Lord?" I had no way of knowing God's plan for my future, but I could have simply trusted that He had one that was being worked out.

God gave me some downtime to think about my long-term career goals. He knew we were about to move to a city within close commuting range of an excellent graduate school of social work. The simple fact that I was chronically discontent about *my* plan not being followed should have told me that I was not accepting *God's* direction.

We all know people who are never happy. I have one friend with a large family income, healthy children, a loving husband, and all the material things a person might want. However, she does not know the pleasure of trusting in God and constantly complains. When someone displeases her she rarely forgives but stores up anger instead. As someone once said, "Being angry at someone is like taking poison yourself and hoping the other person will die." In this case her commitment to being discontented negatively affects her physical, mental, and spiritual health. I pray that one day she will be grateful for and content with God's blessings.

How to Believe that We Can Trust God

Because God is not like us, we can trust Him far more than we can trust one another. Reading Scripture and other books by believers throughout history helps us to know Him by seeing how He has acted. This is crucial, and whenever we neglect this discipline, our faith in God falters. We replace it, of course, by faith in ourselves since we know that others are not to be trusted. I know from experience that this choice again leads to discontent until I come back to Scripture and its promises.

A second approach to trusting God is to lean back and fall into His arms. In the 1960s "sensitivity trainers" taught people about "trust falls." Members of youth groups, therapy groups, and encounter groups stood in front of one another, closed their eyes, and fell into their partner's arms, trusting that they would be caught, a growth experience for many as they learned to trust other people for their welfare. Trust falls have recently become popular again, and YouTube is full of videos of successful and unsuccessful attempts.

This is just a foretaste, however, of the incredible peace we can experience when we fall into God's arms. As we do this, we will find, like the psalmist, that we can rejoice "in the shadow of Your wings" (Psalm 63:7 NKJV). I cannot explain to you how much trusting in God will change your life if you make it a daily habit. But I can tell you how foolish we are to rely on ourselves. He is in control of the entire universe. He is already in charge of our lives; the only question is whether we embrace that and thank Him for leading us or pretend it is not true and struggle against Him.

Why should we rely on God? His perspective is much broader than ours and therefore more reliable. Because He sees more than we do, His timing is perfect. He always works from love, not selfishness. And His ways bring peace rather than discontent. These concepts seem simple, but we will continue to work throughout our earthly lives to understand and believe these truths.

Our Journey Toward Trusting God's Promises

"Lord," I used to ask, "please take away [whatever pain or difficult circumstance I was experiencing]."

"Dear God," I implored, "please give me or someone I love [whatever I thought was needed]."

For years my prayer life centered on such prayers. I treated God like a powerful candy machine: I put in the payment (my prayer) and expected to receive the candy (whatever I wanted to happen or stop happening).

Today my prayers are different: "Lord, I'm trusting you. Prepare me and strengthen me. Encourage me to do what you want me to do in this situation. Teach me what you want me to learn. Help me to be who you want me to be. Let me use your gifts to bless others today. Thank you for caring about me and leading me."

Trusting When Someone You Love Is Hurting

My ability to trust God came in baby steps. I have the most difficulty trusting God's leadership when my children experience pain. For example, when Mark was twelve years old, he contracted Lyme disease from a tick bite. Basketball season was about to start, and Mark had made it to the last phases of try-outs for the middle school team. Overnight he became ill with swollen joints and fever. His doctor said he could not play basketball that year or run for one year in order to allow his knees to heal.

Mark was unhappy. No basketball. No baseball. No just running around for fun. Even if his knees had healed completely (they didn't), he probably would not have made future teams since the team chosen in the seventh grade usually remained intact through high school.

As Mark's mother, I was upset for him. It didn't seem fair that he would get a disease that would stop him from doing what he wanted to do. But God had a different plan: because he could not participate in organized sports, Mark spent his time and energy on music. Mark had begun playing the violin when he was six. When he was banned from sports, he picked up the guitar and bass as well and spent even more time with the violin. He started a rock band, of course, and became concertmaster of his high school orchestra as well as a member of the state honors orchestra. He received a scholarship to attend a summer program in New York with some of the finest violin-ists in the country, and he played in the Princeton orchestra for four years.

Today Mark plays violin every Sunday at his church and belongs to a bluegrass band that plays regularly in the area. Over the years he developed a love for and expertise in record-ing and helps other musicians record their music. He and Carey have written, recorded, and performed many songs together.

Quite obviously, God has given Mark the gift of music, a passion he can follow for the rest of his life. As his earthly mother, I would have done whatever I could to allow him to play basketball, because that is what he wanted when he was twelve. As his heavenly Father, God decreed that Mark would not play basketball, which has benefited him in the long term.

When the kids were young, we taught them that an apol-ogy has two parts: asking forgiveness and admitting culpabil-ity. I remember well the time I apologized to Carey by saying, "I'm sorry; you were right." She didn't let me get away with only half a statement, and prodded me with, "Yes, and you were wrong." In the case of my fears for Mark's happiness, I grow by admitting openly that once again God was right and I was wrong.

When I am tempted to try to change circumstances because someone I love is hurting, I try to remember this situ-ation and many other times when I have been slow to see God's plan. John Sammis sums this up in one of my favorite hymns, "Trust and Obey":

Not a burden we bear,
Not a sorrow we share,
But our toil he doth richly repay;
Not a grief nor a loss,
Not a frown nor a cross,
But is blest if we trust and obey.

Trusting When What You Plan Doesn't Happen

Proverbs 16:9 reminds us, "In his heart a man plans his course, but the Lord determines his steps." Our plans for Carey's college education show the wisdom of this verse. When she received her acceptance to Princeton University in March of 1992, we were very excited for her but concerned at the same time. Although she received a generous scholarship, we would pay more for her schooling there than we would have at the University of Michigan. After meeting with a financial planner, we decided to tighten our belts considerably and use my income primarily for her education.

In June of that year I had my first two heart attacks. By the end of the summer it was obvious that I was too sick to return to full-time teaching. We had enough money saved to send Carey to her first semester and trusted that God would lead us beyond that. Princeton kindly agreed, against their usual practice, to re-evaluate her financial need for the second semester and increased her scholarship enough to allow her to remain for her entire four years. Furthermore, when Mark was admitted to Princeton three years later, the university split the financial need between the two of them, and we essentially sent them both to school for a year for the tuition of one.

Mark and Carey enjoyed outstanding academic experiences at Princeton, but more importantly, they grew spiritually. Both of them became very involved in an excellent evangelical Christian student program there, developed lasting Christian friendships, and thrived in the church they attended (where Mark played music).

I believe that God enabled growth in them through this difficult time in my physical health by providing the finances for them to attend Princeton. We trusted that what He did would be for our good and our children's good, whether allowing them the opportunity to graduate from Princeton or from the University of Michigan. God loves Carey and Mark more than we could ever love them, which is almost unbelievable to us. On earth we will never fully understand His limitless love, but we can trust that His plan is always the right plan.

Trusting When Things Are Not Going Well

You would think that I would have learned this lesson once and for all, but in the fall of 2007, I had a refresher course. I had been especially tired for several months and had recently developed peripheral neuropathy. This nerve dysfunction causes my feet to become alternately numb or burning (sometimes both at the same time) and makes walking more difficult because the nerves in the feet are not clearly communicating the position of my body to my brain. In August I had an unusual bout of dizziness and vertigo. We found that my inner ear had been damaged, and I had permanently lost fifty percent of my balancing ability on my left side.

One major fall re-injured my back, hip, elbow, and wrist on my left side. A month earlier I had surgery on the left wrist after weeks of occupational therapy had not resolved the pain of a nerve disorder called de Quervain's syndrome. Incredibly, during this same time, I also developed trigeminal neuralgia (TN). A blood vessel in my jaw wrapped around a nerve that runs from my ear to my lip. When the vessel contracts, I get lightning-like jolts of pain that feel like someone stabbing me with a hot knife. In the years before modern pain medicines and neurosurgery, TN was nicknamed the suicide disease because so many people committed suicide rather than dealing with excruciating, ongoing pain. I went on a diet of soft foods to minimize the attacks. Concurrently, my stomach muscle stopped processing food at a normal pace, causing pain, gas, and cramping whenever I ate.

One medical problem piled upon another relentlessly. In fact, I didn't want to tell friends and family about what was going on because it seemed truly unbelievable. Just relating the discouraging details of my situation seemed like complaining.

At some point in November I fell apart for about two days. I had lost the motivation to fight. I couldn't eat, use my hands, sit, drive, or walk reliably, and didn't see an end to any of it. Then God showed me that pride was really underneath my attitude of ingratitude. I asked His forgiveness for trying to do it on my own again and for not trusting Him. And once again I asked for the strength to keep on keeping on.

Not surprisingly, I began to be able to cope again. None of the physical problems resolved, but I was better. I began to use a special cane that helps with my balance. I purchased braces for my wrists. I found a great physical therapist and a massage therapist here in my small town. I had radio frequency neurosurgery that burned the nerve in my jaw and temporarily relieved the TN. I began using lidocaine patches to help my back pain and peripheral neuropathy. And I found a probiotic that helps my gut to work better. My friend Maggie sent me lots of good soup recipes. I have made incremental progress in all areas.

But the real progress came in remembering again that *I* am not my body. My *body* can be in really bad shape without *my* being in really bad shape. God has blessed me with a relationship with Him that includes my physical, emotional, and spiritual selves. He loves all of me, and I am in His care. He will never leave me or forsake me: I can trust only that in this world.

What God Asks of Us

When we trust God's promises, His silence for a time should not confuse or frustrate us. Instead, we will understand that He is working even when we cannot see the results of that work and look for His direction even in crisis situations. We can trust because He is faithful.

God asks two things of us. First, He asks that we recognize our brokenness and bring it to Him to be healed. In Psalm

51:17, David states, "The sacrifices of God are a broken spirit; a broken and contrite heart, O God, you will not despise." Why would God want us to have a broken spirit? Because He understands how prideful and selfish we are when we believe that we arrange the universe and make good things happen. We must be broken in order to rely upon His grace for our needs. When we trust, we can know Him better and love Him more fully. We must accept this idea expressed by Eugene Peterson: "We can't save ourselves by pulling on our bootstraps, even when the bootstraps are made of the finest religious leather."

Second, He asks us to give Him our praise at all times. When we understand God's grace we naturally want to praise Him for all of His gifts, including the gift of being able to rely on Him. The writer of Hebrews puts it thus: "Let us continually offer to God a sacrifice of praise—the fruit of lips that confess his name" (Hebrews 13:15). Praising God has a dual purpose in our lives. First, praising Him for His goodness and love reinforces our belief. Second, we teach others about Him when we praise Him.

Learning to trust and praise God is not a once-and-for-all happening, although it becomes more second nature as we practice it. The following prayer comes from my prayer journal and was written after my third heart attack. The beginning of this short prayer illustrates some of my old thinking, and the end shows the new me that the Lord is fashioning.

> August 28, 1993
> Intensive Care Unit
>
> Dear Lord,
> Dr. El Amir has just told me that my chest pain *was* another heart attack and that it was probably due to vasculitis. This means, as you know, that I could have another heart attack at any time, or that the vasculitis could cause a stroke or cut off another organ.

I don't want to die, Lord, and I don't want to be severely disabled, as with a stroke. I want to live to enjoy my grandchildren. I want to travel in a VW microbus. I want to be at my kids' weddings and help Mark choose a college and watch them get their degrees. I want long, quiet walks with Rick and sleeping in his arms on weekend mornings. I want prayer times when I actually feel your hand on my shoulder. I want to write and receive letters from friends. I want to see friends and family come to love and know you. I want to write what you have in mind. I want to praise and worship with other believers. I want to help my parents as they grow older. I want all the prayers in this book answered. I want you to arise and evil to be killed.

My life and times are in your hand. I am not afraid, but I feel very sad. Lord, be close by me and mine as we face this together. Help us to accept *your* plan, whatever it is, and to not let Satan steal our joy tomorrow and every other wonderful day you give us together.

You are our God. Your love for us never ends. Praise the Lord!

In Summary

1. In order to go from self-reliance to God-reliance, we must learn to focus on God, not on ourselves.

2. We do not fully trust God because we think of Him as being like us. Instead, He transcends time, is omniscient, loves us perfectly, exhibits perfect timing, and gives us peaceful solutions. We can trust His plan.

3. God asks two things of us in return: a spirit of brokenness brought to Him for healing and our praise.

Chapter Six

Working with Your Doctors

You will learn:

- to research, formulate, and prioritize questions
- to keep track of your medical care
- to organize your daily medical routines
- to become a real person to your medical team
- to forgive medical mistakes

Do not be wise in your own eyes;
fear the Lord and shun evil.
This will bring health to your body
and nourishment to your bones.

PROVERBS 3:7–8

The nurse rolled a cart into the examining room, the same kind you might normally see carrying medical equipment. But this cart held only paper: huge binders full of my medical chart, including page after page of test results, doctors' notes, X-ray reports, and hospital records. My recent surgeries had finally made my chart so heavy that the medical records department delivered it on wheels rather than trying to carry it by hand.

Rick and I both started to laugh when we saw that information mountain. But behind our laughter was our realization that physicians who are new to my case face a daunting task. Those of us with multiple illnesses expect these doctors to catch up on a complicated and vast history while trying to address a specific current problem, all in the length of a normal office visit!

Carey and I like to work on puzzles. The first step in this process, as anyone knows, is to put together all the edge pieces, fairly easy because they all have one straight edge. The next is to sort the colors, again fun to do because of its simplicity. Finally, you put together pieces of the same color and fit those sections together according to the big picture on the outside of the puzzle box. This is the challenging part, often keeping us up until after bedtime just to "finish this section" or "find where this piece goes."

I respect and admire my medical personnel. They work very hard, and I want to do anything I can do to help them help me. So I do my part: I put the edge pieces into place and sort the colors, giving them the information I have. Then I ask them to put it all together.

Doing Your Homework

Good physicians want to learn everything they can, but none of them can keep up with all the new information available daily to the medical world. My dermatologist, for instance, belongs to a group of doctors who each read several journals and share verbal digests of the articles monthly. We can help them by sharing our own research.

For example, years ago I read an article in *Arthritis Today* magazine (published by the American Arthritis Foundation) about using Omega-3 fatty acids to reduce inflammation. I could not access the original research cited in the article without signing on to a fee-only physician Web site. I asked my good friend Beverly, an internal medicine specialist, to find and print it for me. She read the article, was impressed with its findings, and began to recommend Omega-3 supplementation to patients, friends, and family. The Omega-3 capsules helped me, and my research helped many patients. Shortly afterwards I visited my cardiologist, who unreservedly wrote me a prescription for Omega 3 capsules that has since reduced my inflammation levels and lowered my lipid profile considerably.

Using the Internet

Almost all of us now have access to the Internet, a source of excellent information as well as frustration. You may already be an Internet expert, but I was clueless about it until relatively recently. When you find you have a chronic or serious illness, you should learn to use this resource wisely. Local libraries often offer courses in finding things on the information highway. If yours does not, find a friend who is knowledgeable and ask him or her to spend a few hours educating you.

Separating medical facts from quack theories or medical advertisements can be challenging on the Internet. Most national organizations (such as the Lupus Foundation of America, the American Heart Association, and the American Cancer Society) offer excellent free information on their Web sites. (I have listed Internet resources you can trust in Appendix A, page 217, and at doingwellatbeingsick.com.)

Many doctors, however, shudder when they hear patients begin a sentence with, "I was reading on the Internet..." because of the volume of misinformation posted there. I have even seen doctors looking warily at anything I am carrying that might appear to be printed out from the Internet. Their skepticism is legitimate. Many flashy sites that appear to present valuable information are just portals that eventually push you to buy remedies that are no better than the "snake oil" once sold by traveling peddlers. Be very careful when reading the "research" such links offer. Find out if a reputable organization has created the Web site, and check out the credentials of those researchers quoted. Are the "experts" simply employees of the firm that produces the snake oil? Do they hold degrees in fields appropriate to the disease being studied? For example, I have read "medical advice" from "practitioners" who have doctoral degrees in such fields as education and are not medical professionals at all.

Joining National Organizations

Local and national organizations offer excellent information, including booklets with basic information about your condition. Often their call-in staff will answer your questions or refer you to nationally known experts in the field whom you may consult. Also, staff members may have personal knowledge to share, and they will understand your hopes and fears because they know other people with your specific condition.

Local chapters organize monthly support groups. Some groups clearly project a hopeful, positive attitude. Others seem to be forums for complaining and sharing "poor me" stories. Whether or not you find these helpful will depend on your own natural inclinations, the make-up of the group in your area, and where you are in your understanding and acceptance of your disease. People who are shy and uncomfortable in any group will probably not benefit much from support groups.

Depending upon your needs, you may either feel at home or uncomfortable in your local group. If you are still angry about your diagnosis and find that most of the people in your local group are accepting of or even resigned to theirs, you may not click. On the other hand, if your group is welcoming and supportive of anyone at any stage, you may have found a place in which you can be honest about your feelings and receive encouragement. Group members often help each other by sharing information about new treatments, life changes that have helped them, or the names of good doctors.

Keeping a Log

Keeping a log of your symptoms creates another source of information to share with your physician. Focusing your attention on how your body is feeling every minute of every day would be counterproductive, but keeping track of changes in your physical condition and possible contributing factors to those changes can be helpful to your doctor. You will probably see your physician only every two to three months. He or she relies upon you to report the important changes since your last visit and will benefit from detailed information about your symptoms.

Often when I have told my doctor about a symptom, he has asked, "When did you notice this?" or "What else was going on at the time?" If I had not written it down, I could not answer. We can sometimes more accurately tell our mechanic when we first noticed a certain noise in our engine than we can tell our doctor when a rash appeared.

A log will help you gather pertinent information to share at your appointments. It should include:

- a daily assessment of your condition, on a scale of 1–10 if useful
- a numerical assessment of pain if this is a continuing problem for you

- notations about all changes in medicine or dosages of medicine
- any new symptoms and when they appear or disappear
- major changes in lifestyle; for instance, travel or long-term stressors
- changes in diet, perhaps even a daily food log if appropriate
- changes in function of any organ that has been of concern

Being Ready for Your Appointment

Your medical team is busy, and they want to treat you well. You can help the process by preparing well for your appointments.

Take an Advocate

When you are dealing with a complicated chronic illness, it is crucial to bring someone you trust to the appointment to act as a second pair of eyes and ears while you interact with your physician. You cover a lot of ground in a short period of time during a clinic visit. Often a new piece of information from the doctor will sidetrack the direction you thought the conversation would go. Your advocate can sometimes respond to such information more readily than you might since he or she is not approaching the interview with any preconceived ideas about what should be happening.

Your advocate can also speak for you when you are hesitant to press for something. Most of us have a tendency to defer to our doctors' opinions, even if we do not agree with them completely. If we anticipate that we will be discussing a major issue at a visit, Rick and I discuss it beforehand, allowing me a chance to express my concerns and fears and organize my thoughts. Rick supports me and encourages full exploration of the situation, both in our pre-meeting and at the doctor's visit. Several times he has questioned a course of treatment after

I have silently but not necessarily happily acquiesced to the plan. I always ask Rick before we leave an appointment if he has anything to add, and often his questions have been important in helping us to make decisions about my treatment.

Bring Your Notebook

The next most important thing you can bring to your appointment is a notebook in which you have written any information from your log that you feel will be helpful, as well as the questions you have for the doctor for that visit. (Some people may use a PDA device for this function, but I find it easier to consult and edit a written notebook.) Your notebook should go with you wherever you go medically. Include in your notebook:

- the names, addresses, phone numbers, and fax numbers of all of the physicians you consult, including X-ray departments, MRI people, and pharmacies
- a list of all surgeries you have had with dates and surgeon names
- your insurance information
- a record of the tests you have had and the dates and places they were conducted
- copies of the relevant test results
- photocopies of X-rays, MRIs, and CAT scans and/or reports
- record of your weight and blood pressure from every clinic visit
- record of your blood lipid profiles, if they are being tracked
- copies of the list of questions you have for each visit

As we will discuss more fully in chapter 7, if you are admitted to the hospital, be sure to take your notebook and record the result of every test and doctor's visit there. Tell your family where you keep the notebook in case you are admitted via the emergency room and someone must go to your home to bring it to you. If you are confused or asleep when the doctor visits in the hospital, ask someone to write notes about the visit in the notebook. You can consult these notes later when you are awake and alert.

Request Copies of All Test Results

Because hospitals rely on teams of doctors to provide medical care, patients must act as their own administrative assistants in tracking their test results and diagnostic reports. Recently my friend Catherine learned the importance of asking for copies of such reports and carrying them with you. She is battling cancer and had an MRI to check the progress of her treatment. Several days later Catherine and her husband Chris met with a resident whom she had not seen before. The resident stated that he had reviewed her record for only twenty minutes. He then told the couple that because Catherine had two tumors, one quite large, she had little chance of recovery. He stated the sizes of the tumors and handed her a copy of the report. Catherine and Chris knew of only one tumor and had hoped that chemotherapy was shrinking it. They left the appointment devastated.

Before they met with Catherine's oncologist that afternoon, Catherine and Chris read the MRI report the resident had given them. Although they are not doctors, they easily read the narrative section of the report that stated that she had only one tumor, which had shrunk considerably. The two numbers the resident had mentioned were actually the initial size of the tumor and the current, smaller size. When Chris and Catherine met with the oncologist, he confirmed their reading. The resident had misread the report and delivered bad news when the news was actually excellent. Hours, or perhaps days, of agony had been shortened because Catherine had a copy of the relevant report in her notebook.

I sometimes have had trouble getting copies of these reports, or images, after I leave the MRI, CAT scan, or X-ray departments. Even if you do not anticipate needing copies of the images in the future, ask for copies of the reports to be sent to you before you leave the imaging department. The radiologists always send copies of their reports to the doctor who ordered the tests. When you check in, ask them to mail you a copy at the same time. If they will not do this, notify your doctor's office that you want a copy of the report sent to you when they receive theirs or when you visit the doctor to talk about the results.

If you later need a copy of a report or film and have been unable to get your request filled through the system, go in person to the office that stores the images to fill out the paperwork, and hand it to them. I once had a clerk make an X-ray copy for me while I waited, something I had unsuccessfully been working to get for weeks through phone calls and mailing in forms.

Formulate Questions

If you have multiple medical problems, you will be tempted to ask many questions, which can be overwhelming for both you and the doctor. Once during a visit to my wonderful primary care physician, Dr. McCort, I was in the midst of a lupus flare and suffering from chronic mastoiditis causing dizziness, a torn tendon in my leg, and continuing problems with a disc in my back. I succumbed to the desire to discuss each of these problems, one after another, and we were both exhausted by the end of the visit.

Now I type out a list of questions for each visit and make one copy for myself and one copy for my doctor. I start to make this list several days before my appointment and add to it as I think of things I would like to ask. The day of the appointment I print out the final list and often read it to Rick on our way, asking him for any additions. My doctor often uses my lists to jot notes, which saves her time in dictating her comments after our visit. Making our doctors' lives easier reaps benefits for all of us.

When you make your list, organize the questions in order of importance so that you will be sure to have your most pressing concerns addressed while both you and the doctor are fresh and the doctor is not looking at her watch. This also allows you to dig more deeply into the important questions as your doctor responds to them. For example, if your first priority is finding a new painkiller, you stick with that topic until you have a suitable solution to your concern such as a plan for trying samples or a new prescription.

Dr. Mehmet Oz—prominent heart surgeon, author, and TV host—suggests that you choose three questions to address during each visit. Asking only three questions may be challenging for people with many medical problems, but we should keep working toward this goal. Before you leave your doctor's office, check your list to be sure you asked all of the important questions and understand the answers.

Look at Alternatives

Having a written list and a notebook to write down the results of the discussion also helps you to remember to create with your doctor a plan B. For instance, the doctor might send you for some tests. She will suggest that if the test comes back positive, you will follow plan A. But what happens when her nurse calls and says the test was negative? You are left with the symptoms and no plan for dealing with them, and either need to schedule another visit or wait for the doctor to call you to discuss it again. If possible, work out with your doctor what you will do with a negative result before you leave the office the first time.

You should also ask what alternatives your doctor is considering. One time my mother called to tell us that Dad's doctor had told them Dad was anemic. When I asked for more information, Mom said she didn't know what the doctor thought could be causing the anemia, but Dad was supposed to see another doctor. She didn't know what the other doctor's specialty area was or what he would be looking for. Undoubtedly Dad's doctor had some ideas, but he either didn't communicate them, or, more likely, my parents didn't remember them.

Ask your doctor about his ideas and plans. For instance, today he will be testing for X. If it turns out not to be X, it could be Y or Z. He can tell you what procedures the tests for Y and Z involve, what facility he will use, and approximately when these tests will occur. Then you will both understand the plan and know how the process will probably play out. Be sure to keep copies of the test requisitions your doctor gives you also, in case the scheduling becomes a problem or your paperwork gets lost.

Become partners in this endeavor and use the information well. For example, do not immediately jump to the conclusion that you will need the most difficult, expensive, or painful test when it is actually number five on your doctor's list and will probably never be ordered. Instead, let your doctor know that you appreciate knowing what the plan is and saving time by communicating while you are there rather than through phone calls or additional visits. Many times, for instance, when I have called to get results of a test, I have been able to tell the nurse what the plan should be from those results and expedite the doctor's ordering the next step.

During your doctor's visit, listen well. Write down diagnoses, prescribed medicines and doses, the names of tests, and the names of other doctors to whom she refers you. Ask about the spelling or definitions of any terms you don't understand. This is your time to learn, and the information you glean might save your life one day. For instance, on more than one occasion a pharmacy has given me the wrong medicine. Because I had written down the name of what had been prescribed, I avoided taking something potentially harmful to me.

Once you have listened carefully and taken notes, spend a few minutes reviewing what you have heard. Often, when a medical professional knows a subject well, he or she might explain it in a way that does not make sense to you. Repeat what you think has been said and ask the doctor to amend your understanding of the information or add to it if you have misunderstood something.

For example, when Carey was a toddler and I was still a relatively new mom, she developed a rash for which the pediatrician suggested lukewarm baths with an over-the-counter heavy ointment. I bought this and tried the treatment without success. I called and explained that I had not been able to get the ointment to melt in the water and wondered if warmer water would help. You can imagine how embarrassed I was when the nurse laughed and said the ointment was supposed to be applied to Carey's skin *after* the bath! If I had only checked out what it was I thought I had heard, Carey's rash would have cleared up much sooner.

Be Organized about Medication Refills

You can save some precious time with your physician by being organized about the medication refills you need. Check your pill bottles before your appointment and write down the name, dose, and frequency of any medications you will run out of before your next visit. You can give a list of medicines that you need to have refilled to the nurse or medical assistant who takes your blood pressure and weight and ushers you into an examining room so that he or she can have the prescriptions ready for the doctor to sign.

Some hospitals and clinics now computerize a list of your medications and ask you to check off those you are no longer taking and those you need refilled. This helps all your doctors

Who's Who in the Medical System

Your primary care physician may refer you to a physician who specializes in your particular condition. These are usually doctors who have completed a residency in internal medicine **as well as** a residency in their specialty area, often six to eight years beyond medical school itself.

Specialization:	A Physician Who Treats:
Allergist	allergies to food and environmental allergens
Cardiologist	diseases of the heart such as coronary artery disease or heart failure
Endocrinologist	diseases of the endocrine glands or organs such as diabetes or thyroid disease
Gastroenterologist	diseases of the digestive system such as Crohn's disease and ulcers
Geriatrician	medical problems of the elderly
Gynecologist	women's reproductive problems
Hematologist	blood disorders
Nephrologist	kidney disorders
Neurologist	the nervous system
Oncologist	various types of cancers
Ophthalmologist	medical problems of the eyes
Orthopedic Surgeon	joints that need surgery
Otolaryngologist	medical problems of the ears, nose, and throat
Physical Medicine and Rehabilitation	joint and connective tissue disorders treatable without surgery or post-surgery care

Plastic Surgeon	joints or skin that needs recon- struction
Podiatrist	foot problems such as neuropathy
Psychiatrist	emotional or cognitive difficulties
Radiologist	diseases requiring radiation and reads X-rays, CAT scans, MRIs, and other scans
Rheumatologist	diseases of the joints and muscles such as arthritis and lupus
Urologist	problems of the genitourinary tract

know about medicines prescribed by others, which reduces the chances of dangerous drug interactions. However, I encourage you to keep your own list of medications as well, since computers are not infallible. Remember that you may end up in an emergency room not connected to your primary doctors at some point, and those treating you will need to know immediately what medicines you've taken recently and what your allergies are.

Many of us with chronic illness take numerous medications, and it's nearly a part-time job just keeping track of when we need a new prescription, where the last prescription was filled, what pre-authorization forms our physicians will need to write, and how to appeal when our insurers don't want to pay for a particular medicine. Changing insurers complicates this process, and coordinating several insurances, including Medicare, makes it even more difficult (although those of us with insurance should realize what a blessing this is).

After years of trying to organize all of this through hand-written lists and notebooks, recently I made a master list on my computer to manage this information. I have sections for each of my doctors so that I am not confused about which doctor has prescribed a particular medication. In addition to the names of the medicines and dosage, I list when the prescription was filled, when it can be refilled, where it was filled, how much it costs, and when I will need to get a new prescription from my doctor. I am hopeful that this list of my thirty-something medications will protect me from forgetting to refill a prescription that is crucial to me until the last minute, necessitating rush orders, and perhaps even risking missing a dose.

Helping Your Doctors Remember that Patients Are Human Beings

With all of the pressure placed on our healthcare providers, we can understand their tendency to think of us as cases rather than people. In fact, when I studied psychiatric social work at Yale-New Haven Hospital, I attended many case conferences in which we discussed patients with very little individual identifying information except their symptoms. Unfortunately, we sometimes began to think of a patient as "the obsessive-compulsive" or "the dissociative personality" rather than as a human being with a full life and relationships.

Today's doctors have so much to learn that the human side of their training often gets sidelined in favor of the technical. A few medical schools, however, have decided to train their students to see life from the patient's perspective. The Family Centered Education program, spearheaded by University of Michigan physician Arno Kumagai, pairs medical students with families that live with chronic illness to talk about the impact of illness on the family. Rick and I truly enjoy interacting with these students and feel great that our experiences, good and bad, will help them to be better doctors. I encourage you to use such opportunities to teach your medical team whenever you can.

Practitioners have a limited period in which to identify a patient's presenting problem and pose a solution to it. Medical students are given praise for quickly summarizing a patient's history and current situation. Getting to know more about the patient could be seen as wasting time. But emphasizing efficiency can increase mistakes. Even when the situation is not life threatening, doctors who do not really know their patients often harm them unwittingly.

Years ago I had a friend in suburban Philadelphia who battled diabetes. Because her husband worked downtown, they chose a city hospital for a procedure so that he could visit her more easily. Marjorie found the whirlpool at the hospital very useful and asked the young physician who was doing her predischarge interview how she could obtain a whirlpool for her home use. The doctor responded, "I don't think Medicaid will pay for that." Marjorie's family income was probably higher than this doctor's, but he had made the assumption based on her race that she was a Medicaid patient. Although this mistake didn't harm Marjorie physically, it represented a lifetime continuing struggle against racism that undoubtedly caused her emotional pain and challenged her body's resources.

Becoming Real: How Knowing You Helps Them

Part of our job in doing well as patients is to let our doctors know who we are as human beings. Tell them about yourself: your past, your family, your strengths, your passions, your aspirations. Let them know what kind of person you are. Most doctors will start an appointment by asking how you are. When my doctors ask this, I expand the definition of their question to include my whole self. I may talk briefly about a recent visit from one of my children, share how a writing project is coming, or tell them something I am looking forward to doing.

This will have several effects. First, *doctors will be more likely to listen to you if you are a real person to them.* When I was doing private practice counseling, I had Rick return phone calls from new patients seeking appointments if my hours were already full. I did this because I found it almost impossible to turn down patients who had already told me about their needs. Once I heard about their psychological pain, they became "real" to me rather than just messages on a machine. I often overbooked my life in order to help them. When Rick returned the calls and placed people on a waiting list, he protected our family from overload.

Similarly, if your doctors know you as a real individual, they will more likely react positively to your needs. If they understand that you do not generally overreact to things, for example, they will be more willing to find a place in their schedule for you when you indicate something urgent is happening in your case. If they know that you value attending church regularly and that you have been feeling so ill recently that you have not been to church, they understand the depth of your current sickness, perhaps a better indicator than the ubiquitous one to ten pain scale.

Second, *doctors will be able to fit treatment to your needs more easily when they know you.* When Carey was born, an error in the emergency cesarean delivery caused her to develop pneumonia. She was an otherwise healthy baby weighing a little over nine pounds, but doctors placed her in the newborn special care unit (NSCU) with one- and two-pound preemies so that she could be on oxygen in an Isolette. In that hospital, the NSCU and the obstetrics unit were located on different floors. I was not allowed to leave my room, and the nursing staff would not allow Rick to bring Carey to my floor. After twenty-four hours of labor and a C-section, I could not even hold or feed my baby. I was depressed, angry, and worried about bonding with Carey. I was too tired and medicated to make much fuss, but internally I was fuming.

Several months later, after both Carey and I had healed and were coping well, we made an appointment to see the doctor who headed the NSCU. Rick and I shared our experience and told him that we hoped he would change their policy to keep this from happening to other mothers. He listened carefully and responded well, explaining that Carey had been on room air by late afternoon and could actually have come to my room without much risk. "If I had known you then, I would have brought the baby up to see you myself," he said. But *not* knowing us, he was afraid to risk it. If Carey had caught an infection, we might have sued the hospital, saying they took undue risk in letting her out of NSCU too early. What a sad realization that days of unhappiness and worry could have been avoided if a human connection had been made.

When I became pregnant with Mark three years later, our obstetrician asked if Rick and I would consider being a test couple to challenge the hospital policy that prohibited husbands from staying in the delivery room during cesarean sections. Having delivered Carey, our obstetrician knew us as "real" people, and he was confident we would be a good test case for the policy. Rick did become the first father admitted to a C-section at Yale-New Haven Hospital, and the hospital soon began to allow husbands to attend cesarean births. Only a year later, a prospective mother said to me, "I thought husbands were automatically admitted to cesareans; everyone I know has been." The full story of this amazing transformation in medical policy, told in appendix B, "Our Second Cesarean: Why We Fought to Have My Husband There," shows the potential power of an alliance between the patient and the physician.

In *The Heart Speaks,* well-known cardiologist Dr. Mimi Guarneri talks about learning to see patients as human beings while she was in medical school at Cornell University. An older physician told her class, "If you let patients speak and tell their stories, and you really listen, they'll give you their diagnosis. But if you keep interrupting them and they don't get to tell it, you'll keep ordering tests and lab work and you'll miss the answer that's right in front of you." Any physician who does not learn to listen well will struggle much harder to treat patients well. As people who live with chronic illness, we have unique and frequent opportunities to teach our medical team to listen to us.

We must lead our medical team to realize that we are real people with real needs that they should understand so that they can treat us as whole beings. Sometimes we must expend ourselves for future patients. This is all a part of doing well.

Realizing that Doctors Are Human Beings

We should also learn to listen to our practitioners and respond to them as people. Jesus tells us to love others as ourselves, which requires that we know about them. Too often we don't think about life from our doctors' perspective and assume they don't have any needs. For example, we often ignore their human desire to do well at their work and be appreciated. Our offering a short "thank you" at the end of the visit probably will not let them know how important they are to us or how much we rely on them. Instead, write members of your medical team periodically, specifying how they have changed your life in the past few months or years and thanking them for the sacrifices they make to stay in this difficult field. Bake something delicious for the nurses who faithfully give you your allergy shots, arrange emergency appointments, or order medications for you. Take your medical practitioners and staff cookies when you visit. (Recently one of my doctors said he saw my name on his daily roster and immediately wondered what kind of cookies I would bring that day.) Think about other ways in which you can show your appreciation to these people who support you so well.

If you have a chronic illness like me and have had a lot of medical treatment, probably some of the people involved in your treatment have made mistakes—possibly major ones. In the past I would use some of my valuable energy being angry about these mistakes. How could everyone involved in my treatment, from the surgeons to the people who serve the meals and clean the floors in the hospital, not take my needs seriously? How could they allow themselves to make errors?

But God graciously reminds me that I am human and make mistakes too. No matter how hard we try to do everything perfectly, we cannot. This helps me to forgive honest mistakes and preserve my energy for healing rather than anger. But some people simply do not care much if they mess up. As patients, we must protect ourselves by being alert and teaching these people the importance of "doing well" at their jobs.

We discovered when Carey was born that I am allergic to Demerol, a painkiller commonly used after surgeries. I had been in labor for twenty-four hours and then had C- section surgery. When I was given Demerol, I began to vomit uncontrollably, which was excruciatingly painful.

To prevent this happening again, I always carefully tell everyone in any medical setting that Demerol and I are not a good match. "DEMEROL ALLERGY" is written in red letters on my record and repeated in a sign on my door. Nevertheless, when I was post-surgery for a hysterectomy, a nurse came within six inches of my arm with an injection before I asked her, "That's not Demerol, is it?" She pulled the syringe away and said, "Oh, that's right. You are allergic to it, aren't you?"

This nurse was too tired, distracted, busy, or lazy to give me the attention I needed. I needed her to know that I was allergic to Demerol. I needed to take charge of my own care when she didn't. I needed to forgive her mistake.

Admitting that people simply do make mistakes, unwittingly or through inattention, has led me to know that being angry can harm both me and the person I am angry with. I have rarely seen a positive side of any kind of vengeance. In contrast, I have learned to truly admire people who have been wronged and accept the circumstance with grace and patience.

They are always winners in the situation, no matter the mistake.

For example, my good friend Carol went into the hospital thinking she would be home the next day after an ablation procedure that should have stopped her occasional atrial fibrillation. She woke up to find that the surgeon had not been able to fix the problem and instead had implanted a pacemaker in her heart, a possibility that they had never even discussed. Carol was not prepared at all for this outcome that was probably due, at least in part, to physician error.

When I talked with her that day, she was upset, fearful, and angry—all completely normal reactions. The next day, however, Carol's equilibrium was back. Her physical situation was no different; she would still live with a pacemaker for the rest of her life, but God had blessed her with peace about it. She knew that she must not stress her heart with worry and that she was in God's hands. All the rest was not important compared to these truths. Carol did change doctors, a wise decision, but she has rarely spoken a disparaging word about the man whose error changed her life. I am awed by her example of forgiveness.

Sometimes we should point out an error in an effort to keep another patient from being hurt. For example, when Rick and I talked with the head of the newborn special care unit, we helped him treat his future mothers and babies differently. When such a situation occurs, however, we are charged as followers of Jesus to "[speak] the truth in love" rather than in anger (Ephesians 4:15). Approaching a problem with a loving attitude allows both sides the energy to look at options, which is more productive than digging ourselves into one position or another.

Our medical team is made up of flawed people—just like us. For this reason we should pray with Paul that we may all be "strengthened with all power according to his glorious might so that [we] may have great endurance and patience" (Colossians 1:11). We have been forgiven much by God. Surely we can forgive.

In Summary

1. Do your homework by researching, formulating and prioritizing questions, keeping track of medication needs, and noting symptoms.

2. Help your medical team to realize that you are a human being to aid them in your treatment, and treat them like people also.

3. Be vigilant in monitoring your care and forgiving when others make mistakes.

Chapter Seven

Dealing with Hospitals

You will learn:

- to prepare for emergency room visits
- to help your medical team treat you in the hospital
- to heal as quickly as possible
- to keep an eternal perspective during recovery

From Thee all skill and science flow,
All pity, care, and love.
All calm and courage, faith and hope;
O pour them from above.

CHARLES KINGSLEY

$\mathcal{W}$hen Carey was eight years old, she developed drastic flu-like symptoms, including an uncontrollable high fever. Our small town's one pediatrician was an excellent doctor. He quickly admitted her to the area hospital where he diagnosed her with Reye's syndrome, a rare and potentially lethal infection. The next day he arranged her transfer to the Mott Children's Hospital at the University of Michigan, several hours away. The resident at the large medical center initially thought our country doctor was wrong, but the Center for Disease Control in Atlanta confirmed the Reye's diagnosis. Supported by our praying friends and family, this small-town hospital and doctor worked together with the large medical complex and team to save Carey's life. From this experience we learned an important lesson: good hospitals come in many sizes.

Most people with chronic illness will spend significant time at a hospital, either in emergency situations, for testing, or as an inpatient. While you are healthy, spend some time researching the hospitals in your area. What are their specialty areas, their infection rates, their nurse-to-patient ratio? At which hospitals does your medical team have admitting privileges? Ask your doctors and nurses for their opinions as to the best place for you to be treated if you should need to be hospitalized.

Also check the Internet. The U.S. Department of Health and Human Services rates institutions throughout the country at their Hospital Compare site (*www.hhs.gov*). This site provides, for instance, the success rates of hospitals in treating heart attacks, something you might want to know if you have heart disease. Another Web site, *healthgrades.com*, grades hospitals with one to five stars, similar to ratings for hotels, and gives separate ratings for different situations, such as heart attack care or hip replacement surgery. *U.S. News and World Report* provides an annual summary of the best hospitals in a number of specialties. Investing energy in learning about the facilities available in your geographical area could save your time or even your life later on.

Preparing for Emergencies

Fifty percent of families will visit an emergency room (ER) at least once this year. Some of us go there even more often. (You know you are a regular when you begin to recognize the intake staff.) Preparing for these emergencies could mean the difference between life and death. You should carry with you at all times a kit of pertinent medical information that can be handed to emergency room personnel when you arrive. I keep these papers in a small zip-lock bag in the bottom of my purse, and they have been invaluable a number of times. ER doctors and nurses often compliment my bringing an emergency kit because it allows them to provide better and faster care for me. Be sure your family knows where you keep your kit in case you are unable to speak for yourself at your next ER visit.

For example, once I had chest pain while I was at the University of Michigan Hospital for a physical therapy appointment. Ironically, I thought I had indigestion, just like the ER doctor who misdiagnosed me during my first heart attack. Fortunately, my physical therapist noticed that I was in trouble, took my blood pressure and pulse, and sent me to the ER in a wheelchair.

By this time I was in great pain, but I briefly told the triage nurse about my cardiac history and handed her my kit. You do get moved to the head of the line when you tell the ER staff that you have had three previous heart attacks and are having severe chest pain! They admitted me and saved my life once again. This experience contrasted greatly with the situation in St. Louis when I struggled to tell the ER doctor about my medical history while having a heart attack that he had already decided was indigestion. If you do not want to make your own kit, you can find a form that will cover much of the critical information at *medIDs.com.*

Medication List

You can save precious minutes if you keep a copy of your current medication list in your kit, with your name, date the list was updated, and your birth date at the top. If you receive most of your medical care at one facility, include your registration number there as well. Update the list whenever your doctor adds or subtracts a medicine or changes a dose. Keep copies of your previous medication lists in your notebook or filing system so that you can track medicines you have tried and abandoned, and when your medications or dosages change.

Perhaps the most important part of this package is a list of your allergies. In an emergency, medical personnel work through protocols, or pre-set patterns, to try to save your life. If they do not know you are allergic to a medicine that is part of the protocol, they could give you the medicine. Make sure that you type this section in capital letters and in boldface type so that it can't be missed. Having this information available for those who are treating you could save your life. I have had seven heart attacks and more than a dozen surgeries. By far my most frightening experience, however, was going into anaphylactic shock. During a heart catheterization, the doctors had administered a dye that I am allergic to that caused my throat to swell shut. Struggling to take every breath demands far more faith than living through the pain of a heart attack. If the staff knows your allergies, you can prevent this kind of situation.

Medical History

Take the time to write up a summary of your medical history, including major illnesses, accidents, broken bones, and surgeries. As much as possible, provide dates for these events and diagnoses. Include the names of the doctors and hospitals that treated you. Describe the outcome. For example, "In August 1967 Dr. Smith removed my gall bladder at the University Hospital. I healed well and had no further problems." On a separate sheet inventory all of your surgeries, including dates, hospitals, and surgeons' names. Be sure to include a list of implants in your body, for instance, stents in your arteries or artificial lenses placed during cataract surgery.

At the end of the history include a list of all of your physicians with their specialties, addresses, phone numbers, and fax numbers. This will enable anyone who treats you in an emergency to directly contact someone who has experience with your particular physical condition. Good emergency rooms also use this information to send summaries of your emergency treatment to your physicians, so that they know what has happened to you and how they treated your condition.

Relevant Test Results

I learned after my second heart attack that it is very helpful for physicians to know what my previous heart attacks looked like on an EKG and what my heart looks like on an EKG when it is behaving normally. I now carry copies of my most recent EKG reports in my kit. In addition, I carry a note written on one of my cardiologist's prescription forms that indicates the best treatment for my particular type of heart attack. Having my own physician recommend this treatment saves precious time that might be spent deciding between several approaches to stopping the heart attack.

If you have another chronic illness and regular testing shows its progress, carry that information with you as well. For example, if you are being treated for a slow progressing cancer, you might want to carry a summary of your latest MRI or CAT scan. This could help the ER staff to rule out or implicate the chronic illness in the emergency you are facing.

Medicalert Medallion

The MedicAlert organization provides emergency alert medallions that describe your medical conditions and list your medications to wear either on a necklace or wristband. You can update this information as necessary, and emergency personnel can access your records immediately by phone. This service is helpful if you are unconscious or otherwise unable to communicate.

Staying in the Hospital

Eventually most of us with chronic illnesses will endure a hospital stay. Staying in the hospital will never be fun, but it can be more tolerable with some advance preparation.

Contacting Your Doctor

Before you enter the hospital for surgery or treatment, learn how to contact your doctor or team at any time of the day or night. This may seem strange; you are in the hospital—surely the doctor will be available to you whenever you need him or her. However, this is not usually the case.

Most commonly, while you are in the hospital, you will contact your doctor through your nurse. Since nurses today are generally overworked, this process can be slow or even fail completely. Sometimes nurses determine on their own that your request is not really worth the doctor's time. You should explain as clearly and completely as possible why you believe you need the doctor's input. If the nurse is convinced that there is a real question of treatment that cannot wait until the doctor's next scheduled visit, he or she will be able to contact the doctor quickly through the paging system. Always contact the doctor through the nurse in a non-emergency situation.

Be sure, however, to have with you the phone number of your doctor's office and secretary or office nurse. You can always leave a message that the doctor will receive reliably. If you don't overuse this service, you will find that your doctor will respond when you need him or her. In an emergency, you can also call the paging number of the hospital (which you should also write down in your notebook before your admission to the hospital) and receive an answer in minutes.

The shortage of nursing staff sometimes causes long waiting times in answering call bells. If your request is not urgent, just be patient and someone will eventually respond. When your request is urgent and you are unable to leave your bed, an unanswered bell can frighten you or even threaten your life.

My sister-in-law Michele, for example, was unable to walk her first day after surgery when her IV needle came out of her arm. She was gushing blood, and her painkilling medicine was pouring onto the floor. Frustrated that she could not get an answer from her call button after repeated tries, she called the main phone number of the hospital and asked for the nursing station on her floor. They answered, she told them her situation, and almost immediately someone came to her aid. Since then I always have that main phone number available to me during hospital stays.

Knowing Your Medical Team: Physicians

You will probably see ten to twelve medical practitioners every day in the hospital, ranging from various technicians to senior physicians. Without a written program to consult, how can you tell who's who? Most teaching hospitals assign a team of doctors to handle your case. This will include an *attending physician*, who is an experienced doctor in your field; a third or fourth year *resident* in the specialty area in which you are being treated who will lead the team on the floor; and a rank amateur first- or second-year *medical student* (who will wear a short white coat rather than a long one).

The residents and medical students begin work on July 1 of every year. For the first few weeks they may still be trying to find the copy machine, so if you have an elective procedure, avoid scheduling it for the beginning of July. I once had the misfortune of having a heart attack on July 2, and my assigned medical student almost didn't finish reading my chart before I was released. When I left, he told me, "I've learned so much from you."

Under normal circumstances patients will interact more with medical personnel farther down in rank. For instance, a medical student will be in charge of getting your medical history and interacting with the nurses on the floor. These students are usually exhausted and overwhelmed. They have been thrown into deep water for the first time and are often struggling to keep swimming. They are also, however, tightly monitored by those above them on the team who sign all orders and prescriptions.

Many institutions now use *hospitalists*, or physicians employed by the hospital itself, to follow individual cases and coordinate care for their assigned patients. Hospitalists know the system well, which helps to ensure that patients have the proper tests in a timely manner, that the results are reviewed by specialists, and that all of the appropriate professionals are consulted as to diagnosis and treatment plan. Research shows that when hospitalists coordinate care, patients stay in the hospital for shorter periods of time and hospitals save money, so this trend will probably continue.

Knowing Your Medical Team: Nonphysician Personnel

With so many people coming and going in your room, you can be confused easily about who does what, even when they introduce themselves. I remember the days when RNs all wore highly starched white caps, but today everyone from RNs to maintenance personnel wear brightly colored scrubs, and you may simply not know what their jobs are. Often this leads us to ask the wrong person for something and then wonder why we don't get what we asked for. If you ask the person who is taking your blood sample if you can have pain medication, for example, your request will probably be lost, since that person has nothing to do with medicines. Some hospitals are now trying to help patients differentiate by having the different groups on the medical team wear the same color of scrubs. For example, nurses might wear green, and all the technicians wear yellow. Meanwhile, the following chart may help you to understand the cast of characters in the hospital.

Other Members of Your Medical Team

A large team of professionals supports your physicians in making you well. Knowing what the letters on their badges mean can help you get better care.

Licensed Practical Nurses (LPN) have graduated from a post-high school training program and passed a certification exam. They work under the supervision of RNs or physicians in direct patient care, including monitoring medications and IVs.

Medical Assistants (MA) usually complete a one- or two-year training program at a community college and pass an examination. MAs assist with basic tasks such as taking blood pressure, drawing blood, and preparing patients for exams. Medical assistants never work independently of a physician.

Nurse Practitioners have a master's degree (MNP) and are certified to do basic patient care under the supervision of a physician. Many private practices employ nurse practitioners as primary care staff.

Nurse Aides, sometimes called Certified Nursing Assistants (NA, CNA), often have little or no formal training, although some graduate from certification programs. Aides do unskilled but important tasks such as giving baths, changing beds, and helping in feeding patients.

Nutritionists have studied the relationship between what we eat and how we heal. Cardiologists, for example, often refer patients to a nutritionist for a "heart friendly" diet plan.

Occupational therapists hold master's degrees (*MOT*) and work with patients to increase their functioning and gain independence in their daily lives. Patients who have had strokes or surgeries, for example, often benefit from occupational therapy.

Phlebotomists have completed high school, a two- to four-month career center or medical center training program, and a licensing examination. They draw blood for testing.

Physical therapists hold master's degrees (*MPT*) and focus on exercises to regain range of motion and strength in joints damaged by accidents, surgeries, or disease- and age- related problems. For example, most people undergoing knee surgery will receive several months of physical therapy.

Radiologic Technologists (*RT*) have been trained two to four years post high school and are certified to take X-rays.

Registered Nurses (*RN*) complete at least two years of post-high school education and pass the state exam for RNs. Many hold bachelor's or master's degrees. RNs do patient care, but more often they supervise other LPNs and assistants, consult with physicians, and work as patient advocates. Every floor of the hospital will have one RN who supervises the care, usually known as the charge nurse.

Respiratory Technicians (*RT*) train from two to four years after high school and pass the state exam. They assist patients with breathing problems, including supplying additional oxygen for those in ICUs, ERs, and operating rooms as well as normal hospital rooms.

Social Workers have obtained bachelor's or master's degrees in social work (*BSW, MSW*) and provide psychosocial counseling for persons facing difficult medical or emotional situations. For example, social workers can aid families in adjusting to a family member who becomes disabled or chronically ill.

Gathering Information

Any time we interact with a bureaucracy, one of our major challenges will be transmitting or receiving information. Usually communication problems are the result of human error or misunderstanding, and the results of miscommunication range from momentarily disturbing to actually dangerous. For example, after my first heart attack I had been in the intensive care unit of the St. Louis hospital for several days, accessible to my extended family in another state only through the nurse's station telephone. When my brother Dick made his daily call to check up on me, the nurse said, "Mrs. Wallace is no longer with us." Dick thought that she was telling him politely that I had died. His shock must have been apparent even over the phone wires, because she quickly followed up with, "We transferred her to the cardiac unit today." Today we all laugh at that conversation, but at the time it was not funny! Planning ahead can minimize such miscommunications.

To receive the best care at the hospital, you should understand its daily rhythm. At least once a day, often in the wee hours of the morning, the medical team will do rounds. During rounds the entire group will visit each patient, with the students and residents presenting the patient's progress to the attending physician. The team then determines that day's treatment. The attending physician is the senior member of the team, and he approves, or disapproves, all recommendations. As a practical matter, however, the chief resident assigned to your case will make most of the decisions and direct the members of the team, who are below him in rank.

Hard as it may be for you to think clearly so early in the day, rounds constitute a critical event in your care, and you should be prepared to ask questions, offer suggestions, or make requests at this time. You should direct your questions to the attending physician or the chief resident if you are not satisfied with the answers of your medical student or first-year resident. If at all possible, you should know approximately when your team is coming and have a loved one with you. You may spend some frustrating early hours waiting together for the five minutes you get with the doctors. But just like during office visits, having another person to think through the information being presented and offer questions is often invaluable.

Keep either your regular medical notebook or another notebook or pad of paper on your bedside table. Write down the following:

- the questions you want to ask
- the test results you are given
- the possible plans of action (from 1–5, as in office visits)
- the names of your residents and medical students
- the names of specialists you are referred to
- the names of the nurses, including the charge nurse of each shift
- changes in medication
- changes in symptoms or unusual symptoms
- anything else that you think might be relevant

If you are not able to write, have your loved one or a nursing assistant write things down for you. Recording the treatment plan has often been very helpful to me. For example, because doctors must write out every change in treatment plan, often the nursing staff does not know the latest plan immediately. Once a nurse came in to prep me for a test that the team had decided several hours earlier I was not going to have. Because I knew what the plan was and questioned the prep, I saved time and discomfort.

The notebook can also help family members know what is going on when you are unable to communicate or are confused. If you, or someone who is helping you, write in it any news that you receive, visitors will be able to access the information.

If you have had major surgery, I *strongly suggest* that you arrange to have a friend or relative with you twenty-four hours a day during your first days of recovery, when you might be unable to walk without assistance or are still unclear in your thinking because of painkillers. You can usually arrange for a sleeping chair for a person who is staying with you in your room. Most hospitals today cannot hire enough good direct care personnel, and the staff they have simply do not have time to do all that is asked of them. Having a loved one there to monitor your progress, get you a drink or tissue, wipe your forehead, and ask for professional help when it is needed can be key to your recovery.

My daughter once saved my life by noticing a mistake in medication and insisting that the doctor be called at once. I was on a morphine pump at the time and was unable to monitor my own condition. The resident assigned to my case had misread the dosage for one of my heart medications. The nurse had just given me four times my normal dose when Carey and I realized I had taken three pills too many.

Carey insisted that the staff page the resident who had written the prescription. When he arrived, he told us, "You are taking so many medications, it is hard to keep them straight." Carey suggested to me that if he had a problem with keeping medications straight, he might consider going into plumbing instead of medicine. We did avert a medical disaster, and her humor was just what I needed at a tense moment. Given the overworked state of most medical team members, I encourage you to have someone to cover for you for at least the first day.

Sharing Information

Recent federal legislation (The HIPAA Act of 1996) has made it almost impossible for anyone other than you, the designated patient, to receive your medical information. While HIPAA offers important privacy concerning your condition, this law's requirements can be frustrating and dangerous as well. Once I took my mother for a follow-up appointment with her physician. Her condition had not improved, and the doctor suggested doubling the amount of medication he had prescribed. Because I filled her pill containers for her once a week, I knew that Mom had not been taking the medicine he had already prescribed. A prescription for double the dose would have been useless under the circumstances; a frank discussion with the doctor made a much bigger difference. Again, two heads proved better than one.

I was with my mother when this incident happened, and she gave me permission to speak with the doctor. He would not, however, have been able to talk with me by phone or in person without my mother's permission. Later, in fact, one of the doctor's colleagues refused to discuss my parents' care with me until he had a letter on file from them granting permission. My parents did write a letter for their files asking that my siblings and I be allowed access to their information, which allowed us to talk with their doctors about their symptoms, medications, and course of treatment.

Since my parents were not always reliable in reporting what was going on with their health or in taking their medications, another perspective often helped the physicians and prevented many possible problems for all of us. Once, for instance, my father told his doctor that he didn't really know why he had an appointment with him. Dad had been experiencing severe back pain, but his Alzheimer's disease kept him from remembering this. When I prompted him, he remembered and described the location and severity of the pain.

While you are healthy, decide whom you would like to have access to your medical information, perhaps a spouse, children, a sibling, or a trusted friend. Place a letter on file with all your physicians and with local hospitals you deal with explaining with whom they can share medical informa-

Sample Permission Letter to Access Your Medical Records

DATE: April 8, 0000
FROM: Wendy J. Wallace, DOB 00-00-0000
     U of M Hospital Registration 00000000
TO: Medical Team, University of Michigan
     Hospital/ Chelsea Hospital
RE: Sharing medical records

Please accept this letter as notice that I give permission to you to speak to my husband, Richard Wallace, or to my children, Carey Wallace and Mark Wallace, concerning my medical conditions, test results, or other relevant medical issues. I wish them to have full access to my medical records in order to help with my medical decisions, both now and in the future.

Thank you.

tion. You will rest easier knowing that someone you trust will watch out for you in this way.

You should also have a living will or medical power of attorney stating your end-of-life preferences as clearly as you are able and naming a patient advocate should you be in a physical or mental condition that keeps you from making decisions for yourself. Most hospitals and many doctors' offices have forms that you can use to create a living will, and you can also download various forms from the Internet. A medical power of attorney should be constructed by an attorney, most of whom provide this service for a nominal fee. Be sure that these documents are filed at your local hospital and with your physicians in case of emergency. Adding copies of these documents to your kit could be useful. Advanced planning on your part will help your loved ones in a time that you are not able to help them.

Your In-Hospital Accommodations

Most nurses today are far too busy to fluff your pillows for you or give you a sponge bath. But you can make your stay more comfortable by requesting a private room. Studies have shown repeatedly that people get better faster when they recover in private rooms rather than shared rooms. This only makes sense; it is quieter, there is less chance of infection, and someone visiting or assisting your roommate does not interrupt your rest. Most new hospitals are being built with only private rooms.

Hospitals with shared rooms will not promise you a private room before your surgery or admission, but once you are there, ask for a private room early and repeatedly. Explain to everyone your desire to be in a single room, from the admitting people to the recovery nurse. State your reasons clearly: you are a light sleeper, you have chronic conditions that make it difficult for you to heal, you are worn out already from fighting the disease that you are there to treat. Private rooms cost only a few dollars extra per day, and they are usually not covered by insurance but are a great investment.

Also, if you have a choice, do not choose a room directly opposite the nursing station. Medical staff socializes near the nursing station, and the noise could bother your rest and recuperation.

Some Miscellaneous Ways to Be More Comfortable

Why does the food you eat at the hospital seem so important? I'm not sure. Perhaps because it is the one thing that usually happens on a schedule. Perhaps because we all love to eat. Most hospital food tastes terrible, yet we still look forward to seeing what breakfast, lunch, and dinner will bring. I remember eagerly awaiting my first non-IV meal after colon surgery and being disappointed to find lasagna on my plate, obviously a meal intended for someone else.

Most hospitals give you a menu in advance from which you choose an entrée such as pancakes, eggs, or cereal. What they don't tell you is that there is usually a standardized alternative food list from which you may also order. The alternatives are not fancy fare, but sometimes a plain ham and cheese sandwich sounds much better than an unrecognizable beef ragout. So ask the nutritionist or nursing staff about the hospital's food list.

Another thing hospital staff does not tell you is that if you have had a test for which you have had to fast (called "NPO" in medical jargon) and you arrive back at your room just after lunch has been cleared away, you do not have to wait until dinner to eat. Almost all hospital food services have soups, sandwiches, and fruit available twenty-four hours a day, especially for situations like this. Ask your nurse as soon as you get back to order you a sandwich or other food from this ready-made list.

Recently our medical center installed a Wendy's restaurant right in the hospital, making more enjoyable food available twenty-four hours a day. I often send my family down to get me a Frosty or a chicken salad when the food served in my room leaves something to be desired. If your hospital does not have alternatives, ask your visitors to bring you something from the outside occasionally: a favorite soup from a restaurant you like, for instance. They will enjoy pleasing you, and you will get better sooner with good food in your stomach.

Things to Do While You Are There

If you are a person who loves music as I do, bring a CD or MP3 player, boom box, or radio with you to the hospital, preferably with headphones so that you don't annoy anyone and can listen in the middle of the night if you want to. Choose a few good CDs before you leave home. Listen to things that soothe you when you are trying to relax and things that inspire you when you need inspiration. I often turn to my CDs of classic hymns. Again, much research shows a positive connection between listening to music and healing.

Think about what calms you at home and take whatever you can with you. If you enjoy fiction, bring a good book. If you love old movies, take some DVDs and borrow a portable player from a friend or the hospital if it has that service. If you find comfort in reading Scripture, have your favorite version of the Bible ready. I have spent hours in the hospital just listening to my husband read psalms to me and have a copy of the entire Bible on CD to use when he is not visiting. If doing needlework or knitting soothes you, bring an easy, small project. If you love to scrapbook, bring a box of photos to sort.

As you recover, you may become restless and eager to do things but still physically unable to do so. Walk as much as you are allowed to, in short increments and perhaps even on a schedule. Moderate exercise speeds healing and increases energy. Our lymph system, which is the garbage collection agency of the body, uses our muscles in order to do its work. So take out the garbage regularly, even if you don't feel like it.

A friend of mine once called me when her husband, George, had just had his lung removed. I had undergone this surgery a few years earlier. George didn't want to get out of bed because the pain was wearing him down. His wife was afraid he was giving up, and she knew that exercise was crucial to regaining breathing capacity. I headed to the hospital, found George, exchanged a few words about our situations, and told him I was there to help him take a walk. Perhaps because I wasn't a family member, perhaps because I had lived through this, George got up and allowed me to walk him down the hall. He never balked at exercise again, improved, and lived many more years. Remember George when you feel like staying in bed.

Using Your Recovery Time to Testify to God's Goodness

Often when I am in the hospital a staff member comments on how well I am doing given the particular challenge I am facing at the moment. Such comments provide wonderful opportunities for me to talk about God's gift of grace to me. I am extremely grateful for the excellent medical care I receive. However, I have no doubt that I do well because God loves, strengthens, and encourages me through prayer, Scripture, family, and friends. What a blessing that He then gives me opportunities to tell others about this!

Our time in the hospital can provide opportunities to bring glory to God for His provision for us of this treatment, this hospital, these doctors, and this healing. We can be a walking testimony to His grace in this life and to our hope in the next.

At the same time, give yourself permission to have days when you don't feel like being a testimony. In fact, you may have days when you doubt the entire process of healing is worth the energy you are spending on it. These days may result from medication changes. Sometimes they reflect your pain level. Occasionally you won't be able to find any reason for them. But your heart knows that these moods will pass, so just wait them out and begin again the next day.

Remember that your recovery period will be short compared to the rest of your life. You will have to work your way back to your normal routine slowly. Be patient and thank God for the opportunity to do this work. You will heal more quickly and bless your friends and family while doing so.

In Summary

1. Have an emergency information kit with you at all times.

2. If you have advance notice, prepare for your stay in the hospital to help your medical team in treating you and to heal as quickly as possible.

3. Keep an eternal perspective when recovering from illness.

Chapter Eight

Living with Pain

You will learn:

- to plan ahead to minimize pain
- to reduce pain through regular care
- to "treat" yourself daily
- to accomplish something even when in pain
- to hang on at the end of your rope
- to begin to allow the pain to bring you closer to God

Hear my prayer, O Lord;
let my cry for help come to you.
Do not hide your face from me
when I am in distress.
Turn your ear to me;
when I call, answer me quickly.

PSALM 102:1–2

Oh, I'm sorry. I didn't realize you were asleep." My college roommate had once again barged into our very small dorm room, flipped on the light, and awakened me. I will never understand why she was surprised time after time that I was sleeping when the room was dark and dorm-closing time had passed. She was a sweetheart but had never shared a room before. She simply didn't know how to do it.

Chronic pain resembles a roommate we get when we either can't afford rent on our own or a school randomly assigns us someone to live with. Although roommates often bring much joy into our lives, some of them may also wake us at odd times, sap our energy with their problems, become a constant presence we can't retreat from, or even eat our groceries without helping to pay for them.

Pain does all this and more: pain keeps us awake, exhausting us and keeping us from the things we really want to do; pain allows us no escape; and pain often eats our time and money without any payoff. Chronic pain becomes an almost human presence. We either become angry, or we learn to live with it. I am still friends with my college roommate; even forty-five years later, we care about each other. Pain has not become my friend, but I have learned to live with it.

The Public Face of Pain

People will have trouble understanding that you have ups and downs in your wellness. Your good friends will know because they see you often and have lived through changes with you. The general public never will.

I have learned not to care much about the opinion of the general public. When someone sees me out walking or driving with Rick, they assume that I am okay and that they can ask me to do other things such as chair a committee at church or teach a seminar. I often receive puzzled reactions when I explain that this is not a good time for me to commit to something.

When intense, chronic pain moves in to stay in your life, no two days will be alike for you. You cannot wholeheartedly agree to a course of action days or weeks from now because, frankly, you don't know what kind of day that will be for you. These ups and downs may occur on the same day. I frequently go to the grocery store and see produce or other food products that stir ideas for great meals. I buy the products enthusiastically and take them home, where I unload them from the car and unpack them from the bags. By the time I have finished this process, which is routine for most people, I am exhausted, sore, and need a nap. While resting, I try to think of something easy but healthy I can make for dinner. All thoughts of a special meal are gone. Perhaps I will make the fancy meal another day. Perhaps I will end up throwing out that produce when it goes limp. I will not know until it happens.

Planning Ahead

Planning ahead helps me cope with such unexpected pain and weariness. Even more than most people, people with chronic pain must be organized in order to cope with our lives. Planning can be the difference between lives of contentment and lives of frustration for us and our loved ones.

Lists of Lists

As I mentioned in chapter 3, I keep a notebook divided into three sections with a long-term list, a medium-term list, and a short-term list. I choose my daily tasks from the short-term list. The medium-term list includes those things that I will need to do in the near future. The long-term list shows activities I would really like to do but may or may not ever get to.

When we are planning something major like a family party or a long trip, I may make an entire notebook devoted to that event. Again, I divide the notebook into sections based on when tasks need to be completed. Having a place to write down everything I need to do lowers my anxiety level since I don't have to keep all of these things in my head at once.

Daily Lists

Every night before I go to bed I make a one-page list for the next day using the short-term section of my notebook. I sleep better knowing what I hope to do the next day. My daily list includes those things I honestly think I can accomplish with the most pressing tasks at the beginning. At least once a week I check my medium- and long-term lists to include tasks that may have become urgent.

I don't always finish my daily list. Sometimes I barely get it started. But knowing my priorities keeps me from wasting time and gives me a great sense of accomplishment when I cross off tasks.

Grocery and Meal Lists

I keep my grocery list in a spiral-bound stenographer's notebook in the kitchen cupboard and add items to it when I open the last jar or box of something. When I am really organized, I make a monthly calendar of dinner menus and check it before grocery shopping so that I have all the ingredients I will need for the upcoming week. I also keep a written list of easy but healthy meals I can make from ingredients I always have on hand. This sounds simple, but when I am really tired or sore I have trouble thinking creatively, let alone healthily.

On the cover of the notebook I have written, "Insist on light bags." I don't enjoy being different. I really would like to go through the checkout line just like everyone else, heft my bags into the car and out of it, and throw around five-pound bags of flour as if they were ping-pong balls. However, when I try this I spend sleepless nights with pain that only strong drugs can relieve because I've over-stressed my joints.

Most grocery clerks do not believe me when I ask them to make the bags light. Some baggers simply don't understand the concept. Others seem to resent my asking for special treatment. To protect myself, I check what they do as they do it. If I cannot easily lift the bag they put into my cart, I take another bag from their bag stand and unload some of what they have put into the first bag until there are two light bags. When they see me do this, they understand that I am serious about the weight of bag I can lift.

Find grocery clerks who appreciate your situation, and try to stick with them. Remind them every time, however, and thank them for their extra effort. Even the most understanding workers can't be expected to remember every need. And apply this principle to other recurring situations in which you can plan to avoid pain. These days Rick or a friend usually drives me when I go shopping, and my canes preclude my carrying grocery bags for myself, but nobody should lift bags that are too heavy, and I still benefit from remembering to ask for what my body needs.

Rainy Day Lists

When I was a child, if I got bored on a rainy day I threw a sheet over a table and created a fort, clubhouse, secret country, or new planet. Hours later I would emerge satisfied rather than frustrated that the rain had kept me from going outside.

As adults, we can do this when we face days of pain. At times pain and the fatigue that often comes with it prevent us from doing even simple things we love like needlework, woodworking, or playing an instrument, just as the rain forced us inside when we were young. Keep a list, perhaps in your list book, of things you can do when you can't do anything else. My rainy-day list includes sorting through boxes of photos in the cupboard and basement or phoning friends whom I am always thinking of but haven't talked to in a long time.

If you do not prepare for your rainy days, your exhaustion will probably keep you from thinking about how to cope with them. Having a list to choose from will keep you in the proactive rather than reactive mode and help you to feel satisfied rather than frustrated while you wait to feel better.

Lists for Getting Away

Planning ahead is especially crucial when you are anticipating a real change in routine such as visiting a relative's house for a holiday afternoon or even going on vacation. Don't feel embarrassed to take your special sitting pillows or food with you to the family dinner. Other people will be comfortable if you are comfortable, and they can learn something about coping with illness and relying on God from watching you do it gracefully. They would much rather make special arrangements for you than have you pretend that your back wasn't sore in that straight-backed chair of Aunt Margaret's.

When planning a longer trip, get out a notebook several weeks in advance and write in it all the things you use every day. Then list all the things you need so that you can escape home. You can even have one list for warm weather and one for cold. I keep my list on the computer so that I can print it out and check off the items while packing my suitcase at both ends of the trip. This keeps me from forgetting a medication or inhaler or special pillow at home as I prepare for my trip or leaving it at my daughter's house six hundred miles away when I return home.

Begin making your list well before your trip because you may use some things only rarely but have difficulty finding them away from home if you need them. For example, I have one medicine that I use less than once a month, but if I don't take it, I can be in pain for hours. If I were packing at the last minute, I might forget to take this along since I don't keep it with my daily medications. If you are like me, your entire carry-on bag may hold only medicines, patches, creams, and appliances, but your time away from everyday life will be worth the planning and packing.

Packing List for Wendy

Wedge pillow and long pillow
Head pillow and green pillows
Gray pillow
Pillowcase and fleece blanket
Sleeping pills
Eye drops and eye gel
Flonase and Flovent
Astelin
Lidocaine patches
Paper tape
Nitrodur patches
Sportscreme
Lip moisturizer
SI Belt
Exercise sheets

Daily activity sheets
Ring splints
Hand splints
Elbow pads
Glasses case
Noise machine
Orthotics
Sleeping braces
Round and flat brushes
Hair dryer
Face cream

Alcohol pads
Tweezers
Tylenol
Night light
Two kinds of soap
Two kinds of shampoo
Scalp medicine
Band-Aids
Antibiotic cream
All meds in pill containers
Nitroglycerin spray
Multidophilus w/ cooler pack
Lovaza
Sublingual nitroglycerin 2.5
Simethicone, chewable and regular
Citrucel, spoon, and cup
Sinus rinse packets and bottle
Distilled water
Cell phone
Medical history and med list
Non-latex gloves
Bible
Reading book
Prayer list
Devotionals
Hat, gloves, coat, scarf

Sunscreen	Sunglasses and sun hat
Toiletry bag	Humidifier?
Electric toothbrush	Air cleaner?
Vaseline	Bottles of juice and water
A&D Ointment	Underwear, nightgown, robe,
Any extra meds I'm on	Slippers, swimsuit, slacks,
	tops,sweater, dress, shoes,
	socks, nylons

Caring for Your Body Every Day

Taking good care of your body every day alleviates pain in chronic illness. We will all have times when we do a better or worse job of this, but our goal should be to develop habits that contribute to wellness.

Medical Checklists

Once a week I fill compartmentalized pill containers with the medicines I take with my meals and at bedtime. However, I have breathing medicines, creams, patches, exercises, and other things designed to make me mobile which do not fit into containers. For these I have developed a medical checklist that I consult and check off several times each day.

Forgetting my medical routines can create havoc in my life. For example, I once made a trip to the emergency room because I forgot to put on my nitroglycerin patch and then physically overworked. Another time I failed to rinse and brush out my mouth after using my steroid asthma inhaler and developed a case of thrush that lasted weeks, even with medication. I have frequently ended the day with some part of me sore only to realize that I forgot to ice it or put cream on it or exercise it. Using my checklist minimizes these omissions and helps me to do well.

TASKS	Mon	Tue	Wed	Thu	Fri	Sat	Sun
Mornings							
Back exercises							
Neck exercises							
Shower exercises							
Wrist exercises							
Elbow exercises							
Ankle/foot exercises							
Balance & wall exercises							
Pre-breakfast meds							
Breakfast meds							
Omega Threes							
Nitro patch							
Flovent and rinse							
Eye drops							
Astelin							
Treadmill							
Metamucil							
Mid-day							
Prayer & Bible							
Ice back							
Treadmill							
Metamucil							
Lunch meds							
Align							
Eye drops							
Wall ex & nap							

TASKS	Mon	Tue	Wed	Thu	Fri	Sat	Sun
Evenings							
Back exercises							
Wrist exercises							
Elbow exercises							
Ankle exercises							
Balance & wall exercises							
Pre-dinner meds							
Dinner meds							
Omega Threes							
Flovent and rinse							
Eye gel							
Flonase							
Ice back							
Bedtime meds							
Remove patch							
Nasal rinse							
Patches & creams							
Heat back							

Eating Well

We don't have to eat only organic vegetables to eat well. In fact, the vast majority of us will sometimes find ourselves eating fast food. Planning ahead can make most of our meals help us to be well. For example, I find that making a monthly calendar of dinner menus spurs me to try new healthy recipes. This practice has the added benefit of not having to decide every day what to cook and shortening the process of making a weekly grocery list, either for you or someone else. New resources abound for good eating, including magazines such as *Cooking Light* and *Eating Well*. Every bookstore offers healthy food cookbooks that could keep your menus changing for years.

Drinking Up

Keeping our bodies hydrated is crucial as well. Water flushes out toxins from our systems and carries vitamins, minerals, and other nutrients to all our cells. Without enough water our digestive systems do not work properly and our breathing apparatus malfunctions.

Most of us should replace about eight cups of fluid per day that we lose through urination, breathing, and sweating. The National Institute of Medicine guidelines suggest that men drink thirteen cups of water every day and women nine cups. Additional water should be added if you are exercising vigorously, sweating from heat, or sick with a virus or infection. Even mild dehydration can cause fatigue, muscle weakness, dizziness, and headache. In fact, some doctors hypothesize that simple dehydration causes most everyday headaches.

Check your water's purity and filter it until it is good for you. Then drink lots of it. Keep your water glass out on the table or counter all day to remind you to drink. Your body will thank you.

Supplements

Talk with your doctors about vitamins, minerals, and supplements that might help your particular condition and take those you choose together daily. Many great resources address these topics, including *www.realage.com*, which provides a short questionnaire and then offers you specific suggestions as to diet and supplements you might want to take. The Web site that accompanies this book, *www.doingwellatbeingsick.com*, will give you basic information about nutrition and supplementation to start your research.

Medications

Take your medications regularly, even those you don't really want to take. For years I resisted using pain medicines, thinking that one day I might really need them and should wait until then. I have found this was a foolish assumption. In fact, the pain reaction is such that we experience pain more intensely if we let it grow beyond a manageable level. You should always take your pain medication before the pain becomes too severe.

Similarly, medications that help you sleep can be invaluable in doing well. No physical condition will do anything but get worse without rest. Most of us should spend about one-third of our hours in reconstructing and rehabilitating our bodies through sleep. Fatigue magnifies pain, stresses the entire body, and makes us worse. Our bodies heal as we sleep, and sometimes we need medicines to help us do this. What a great feeling to wake up rested!

Doing Special Things

Chronic illness will change our lives. However, we should take stock of activities that are important to us and do all in our power to make them happen. I believe that God has given us talents and passions, and He delights in seeing us use and enjoy them. We are, often in a real sense, fighting to stay alive in this world. We need things we love to do to make this life worth living. Some of these special things may be once-in-a-lifetime events while others could be daily occurrences.

Rick and I are musicians. During our forty-four years together we have loved to play classic jazz duos with Rick on trombone and me on piano. We play music together almost every day and have found that most stress in our lives can be immediately alleviated by a good dose of George Gershwin, Hoagy Carmichael, Richard Rodgers, and other jazz greats.

For years we played oldies for sing-a-longs at our local nursing home, but Rick's dream had always been to do a gig at a restaurant. Last fall we were delighted to be asked to play the "jazzy brunch" at a local fine dining restaurant. We immediately started to practice for longer sessions so that my ability to sit and play would increase. We chose a set list of favorite songs to stretch out through the almost three hours we would be playing.

And then, a week before our debut, my lupus flared. I could hardly sit down; my joints were swollen; I was exhausted. I rested, ate well, increased my water consumption, and generally did everything I could to make myself well. Finally I talked with my primary care physician. After I told her how important this was to us, she said, "Double your medicine for a few days and then take this other medicine, because you will need it the day after." And that is just what I did.

Along with our electronic keyboard, we took an orthopedic office chair to the restaurant. It was outfitted with two sitting pillows. I placed anti-inflammatory patches on all my major joints and slathered creams on the rest of my muscles. I wore braces on my knees, elbows, and wrists, as well as the ring splints I use for my fingers. Underneath my fancy clothes, I was outfitted like an injured player going in to get the touchdown and save the reputation of the old home team.

Many friends and family came, and our afternoon was filled with joy and laughter. Rick and I had *so much fun* that we are still talking about it months later. Of course I was sore afterward—almost anybody would be. Playing your heart out for that long is physically taxing. But the soreness was well worth it.

The audience liked us so much that the restaurant asked us to come back for a return engagement, which we gladly signed up for. But as that date approached, we realized that this time no amount of bracing and patching would make it possible for me to play. Rick talked with the manager, who assured him that she will welcome us back again whenever I am able. Continuing problems have reinforced our decision. Discretion at this point was the better part of valor.

Don't endanger your long-term health in order to participate in something. But as much as possible, do those special things, even if they require extraordinary measures. The healing power of the joy you experience and bring to others will outweigh the temporary pain.

Having Some Treats Every Day

Fun should never be reserved for someday. When you make your daily list, be sure to include some special treats for yourself. Only you know what you will look forward to. I used to love taking baths. Now I don't easily get in and out of the tub, but playing a good Chopin sonata lifts my spirit every time.

I love to bake but can't eat many baked goods, so I have discovered the joy of baking for others. Almost every week I bake treats for Rick's college students. I enjoy the baking, and they enjoy the eating—a great deal for everyone. (Some people think my cookies account for his great classroom ratings; I think his teaching stands on its own merits.)

Our son Mark is also a musician. His day job is strictly suit and tie, business lunches, long hours, presentations, and stress. At night he puts on blue jeans and a white shirt and plays fiddle in the bluegrass band Black Jake and the Carnies. Mark loves playing with the Carnies. He enjoys playing violin and guitar in church every week also, but the abandon and good times the Carnies share are his treat.

Because disability often draws our daily boundaries tightly, we must actively plan our treats. Go for a walk on your favorite nature trail. Make your grandmother's lemon pudding cake. Work in your woodshop on something you don't need. Look ahead to create these times that can keep you from despairing in difficult moments.

Praying When You Feel Like Giving Up

Even with the best-laid plans, there will still be times when we feel like giving up. The combination of pain, multiple things going wrong at once, and sadness from not seeing positive results eventually leads us all to days of deep discouragement. We want to demand either that God cure us immediately or release us from this life.

As I mentioned, I pray every morning before I get out of bed and frequently during the day. Sometimes I write in a prayer journal, and an entry from one day in 1994 shows this kind of struggle.

Dear God,

> Please give me strength and faith. The fear comes and goes, but sometimes I am overwhelmed. I know it is silly to be frightened. I am held in the palm of your hand.
>
> I realized this morning that my prayer should not be, "Lord, keep me in your sight today," but rather, "Lord, keep me watching you today."
>
> I am growing so much through the pain, and love is showered on me. I thank you, Lord, for amazing certainty in the midst of chaos. You are always there.
>
> So once again I ask only for growing faith and patience.

This, Too, Shall Pass

Remembering that these times are transitory gets us through them. Feelings come and go, but God's truths are eternal. He promises to never leave us or forsake us (Deuteronomy

31:6). He tells us that He shares our pain and will ultimately wipe away every tear from our eyes (Revelation 21:4). He walks with us through the valley of the shadow of death, not sending us through it on our own (Psalm 23:4). He is available to us constantly, inviting us to call upon Him (Psalm 145:18).

Job's wife was not the first nor will she be the last to say, "Curse God and die!" We must learn to tune out this bad advice and to refute it if appropriate. Job knew the truth and held out for it against friends and family. Eventually they all understood and Job was able to say:

I know that you can do all things;
   no plan of yours can be thwarted...
Surely I spoke of things I did not understand,
   things too wonderful for me to know...
My ears had heard of you
   but now my eyes have seen you (Job 42:1–3, 5).

We are not complete at birth or at age eighteen, thank God! We are always in process and will be until we reach heaven. God wants us to know and enjoy Him. Sometimes pain drives us to His side.

Pain Brings Us Closer to God

I try never to forget that pain continues to bring me to God. Many of us pray when we are desperate. We really understand that God is God and we are not when we are in horrible circumstances. We humble ourselves before the Lord of the universe when we know how out of control we are. We petition Him for grace when we are beyond any human help.

In an article in the February 2010 issue of *In Touch* magazine, Charles Stanley wonderfully expresses the positive outcome of such situations: "At times God takes the people He uses and places them in impossible situations—in that way, they discover that He is faithful. We may prefer to acquire faith by reading a book, but the Lord knows that the best classroom is a place of utter helplessness."

You need to give yourself permission to have bad moments—even bad days. They happen. But never assume they will become your norm from then on. Instead, thank God for that day and pray for more clearness of His light in the next day.

Dangling at the End of Your Rope

We've all heard the old saying that when you come to the end of your rope, you should tie a knot. Clever, but I never understood it exactly. How do you tie a knot with one hand while holding on to the end of a rope with the other hand? And what kind of a knot does one tie under those circumstances?

We all have these times, especially those of us who deal with pain on a daily basis. Sometimes I simply hold on, knowing that help will arrive. Sometimes I stretch out my feet and realize that ground is only a few inches away. Sometimes I decide to just swing and sing.

Katie, a special young woman who blesses my life, recently e-mailed me an important question: "How, when you're at home and not feeling well, do you find days or times that feed your soul?" I have not written her back yet, but I have been thinking about the answer. What practical things do I routinely do to bring me back to wholeness in the midst of physical trials?

Showing Up

First, I always get up. Just moving, taking a shower, dressing in clothes I'm not embarrassed to be seen in, eating breakfast, and walking a few minutes outside, inside, or on the treadmill make the day seem livable. Everything I manage to do leads to something else I can manage to do, building a sense of empowerment rather than of defeat.

Except on days in which I am seriously ill or recovering from surgery, I do these things whether or not I feel like doing them. I never consider simply staying in bed, not eating, or not getting dressed, because I know that this inaction would lead to spiraling down rather than up. Moving in a positive direction, in and of itself, creates positive emotions.

Psychological studies clearly show that behavior usually precedes attitude, whether positive or negative. For example, people who have been hospitalized for clinical depression often will be labeled better by other patients and staff members before they themselves feel better. Days later, after the patients acknowledge that they are making progress, those around them will place the date of recovery at days or weeks earlier.

Similarly, we have all been in social situations where we act as if nothing is bothering us when we are actually having a hard time. We pretend to be fine because we don't want to bring attention to ourselves or distress to those around us. Sometimes we end up enjoying the camaraderie so much that we may almost forget what is bothering us. So showing up is very important in the battle.

Action Plan

Second, I usually do something physical. Exercise produces endorphins, and, simply stated, endorphins make us feel better. When we move, our spirits rise. Sitting still challenges us emotionally as well as physically. I can manage walking only in short stretches, but I walk almost every day. I never jog, and I am not positive that my treadmill can go over two miles per hour. But walking doesn't require me to be an athlete, just committed to moving my body. Walking outside brings the added benefit of exposing me to the sun, which improves my spirit and protects me from major diseases with its natural vitamin D.

What Can You Do?

Third, I reach out to help others. On days that I am just barely hanging on myself, I cannot make a meal to take to a shut-in or offer to take a friend's children for the day, but I can make a phone call or write a note. Invariably I feel better going outside of myself to encourage someone else on the journey. Jesus told us to love one another, not just as a practical way to sustain Christian community but also because loving others leads to our own spiritual, emotional, and physical wholeness.

Others Have Been Here

Fourth, I use the wisdom of other Christians to keep me on track. I listen to mix tapes of hymns and praise songs to remind me of theological truths and blessings I may forget on days when my body is not functioning well. I post Scripture cards on the bulletin board next to the phone. I read Oswald Chambers' *My Utmost for His Highest* every day. We read through the entire Bible every year in daily readings. I prepare for our weekly small-group Bible study during the week. I keep a copy of Colossians 1 on my dresser and pray it for myself and my loved ones every day as I am dressing and doing some of my exercises. I have read the book of Psalms all the way through a number of times when I've been desperate for God's presence in pain. I sing through my hymnal, thinking about the lives of the saints who wrote the words that still inspire hundreds of years later.

You Are Not Alone

Finally, I have a few friends I can call when I am discouraged. I tell them I am in bad shape that day and ask them to pray for me. Choose these friends well: you will not easily survive the bad days without them, and you will want to share the great days with them.

Learning to Live With It

The hilarious film, *Grumpy Old Men*, details the adventures of Max and John, two octogenarians with their fair share of aches and pains. In one scene, Max shares the story of a mutual friend. "Did you hear about Old Billy Henshell? He was killed in a car crash. Head on collision with a freight truck. Cleared his car straight over the bridge into the Mississippi."

"Lucky guy," John immediately replies.

"You bet," Max responds.

Most of us who live with chronic pain can relate to Max and John's response. Rather than become more incapacitated, we might welcome a quick and clean end to this life and entrance into the one to come. I have consciously wished that I would one day die quickly rather than by inches. But we must remember that we are in this for the long haul, whatever time and circumstances bring. God knows our deepest needs and desires. We must change our attitudes and behaviors according to this knowledge with the help of the Holy Spirit.

Obviously, God could have created a different plan for bringing us to His throne and making us complete human beings rather than having us learn to live with physical and emotional pain. Others, however, often see people who have been insulated from pain as "spoiled." They may be unable to form good relationships because they have trouble thinking about others' needs.

In contrast, most of the "saints" in this world have experienced great pain in their lives. Their pain often teaches them to rely on God. In addition, pain speaks to the human condition, helping us to understand and empathize with one another.

I have shared hospital rooms with many people and experienced firsthand both "saints" and "spoiled." One of my most demanding roommates had never been in the hospital before. She was not very ill but was determined to be cared for constantly. Her needs seemed paramount, and she showed no patience whatsoever.

In contrast, another of my roommates was a young woman who traveled hundreds of miles every month for treatment of a fatal illness she had been battling for years. Susie showed great interest in me and everyone else she came in contact with. When she was feeling well, she busied herself in trying to help me and the nurses. Susie always had a positive word to share and enjoyed every day we spent together. Through her own pain and suffering, she had gained an appreciation for life and unusual desire to serve others.

I continue to learn the lessons God wants me to master concerning living with pain and disability. Recently, a complication of my lupus caused me to lose fifty percent of my ability to balance on my left side. I am constantly dizzy and have had a number of falls as a result. To steal the motto of the U-Haul company, standing up and going across a room now sometimes seems an "adventure in moving" for me.

After extensive testing I went to see the otolaryngologist, hopeful that some medicine or procedure would be a help. But Dr. Telian explained that the damage is irreversible. On the way home, I fumed to Rick that once more a doctor had told me I would have to "learn to live with" a disability. Even as I spoke, I realized that the important part of that phrase was that I would still be living! Learning to live with something means continuing life, continuing relationships, continuing opportunities to know and serve God. Wonderful!

Living with pain involves more than somehow being able to cope. We must accept that God is in control whatever happens. We must understand that life is worth living when we have the right attitude. We must use our gifts to the utmost. We must bless others with our lives however we can.

Every morning before I get out of bed, I thank God for another day of life here and ask Him to let me be a blessing to someone. When I am in bed at night, I thank Him for the opportunities He gave me that day. When you feel like giving up, pray that God will again give you a heart full of gladness and gratitude. And while you are still here, take steps to make your days as pain-free and full of praise as they can be.

In Summary

1. Realize that the public will never really understand the cyclical nature of your pain and how it affects your life.

2. Thinking ahead will enable you to work with your pain to have as complete a life as possible.

3. Taking regular care of yourself, including taking medication for pain and sleep, can be crucial to dealing with chronic illness.

4. Doing special things may require planning and sacrifice, but they are almost always worth the effort.

5. Be sure to treat yourself daily. Life should not center on needs alone.

6. Plan for days when you are debilitated by pain so that you will still have a sense of accomplishment.

7. Inevitably you will have days when you feel like giving up. Realize that they will pass and that they can bring you closer to God.

8. When you are at the end of your rope, keep a regular routine, reach out to others, study the written wisdom of those who have lived through these valleys before you, and realize that you are never alone in this experience.

9. Allow God to teach you how to live well.

Chapter Nine

Changing Life Attitudes

You will learn:

- to distinguish between happiness and contentment
- to believe in God's provision
- to avoid despair by focusing on others
- to trust the future to God and thank Him for the present
- to adjust to the seasons of life
- to lighten your load
- to accept yourself as you are and others as they are

I have learned the secret of being content in any and every situation.

Philippians 4:12

$\mathcal{F}$ive drive-in windows at the bank, and all of them had lines! How was I going to finish my errands and get home in time to make dinner? I could feel my blood pressure rise.

When our bodies are working well, we often allow inconsequential events to use some of our energy. Slow checkout clerks annoy us. We are angry when a store doesn't have a piece of clothing we wanted to buy. Even discovering that we have recorded the wrong TV program knocks us off balance. Once we have been forced to realize our mortality due to serious illness, however, little things seem even littler, and we are more likely to enjoy today rather than spend it complaining.

Modern society teaches us some myths that are antithetical to living well with chronic or serious illness. These include:

1. I am *owed* a happy and healthy life.
2. I am in charge of my own life.
3. What happens in my daily life is what is important, often to the exclusion of my relationship to God and to others in my life.
4. This life is what counts.

When we buy into these myths, we become even more frustrated by life with illness. One of our tasks in learning to live well is to learn the truths that will set us free to be well in sickness.

Society's Myths vs. God's Truths

I Want to Be Happy

God's basic plan for us here on earth is to learn to know and love Him. Based on this love, we learn to love others. This contrasts sharply with the present philosophy expressed in a popular song: "All I want to do is have some fun, and I've got a feeling I'm not the only one."

We are arguably the most spoiled people of all time. The average American family spent 200 percent more on their children in 2005 than they did in 1995, even accounting for inflation. The average household spends over a thousand dollars on Christmas presents. Middle class children feel underprivileged if they don't have their own cell phones. Many families have more than one television set and multiple vehicles. Although poverty is a serious problem in the United States, large numbers of our children are not being sold into slavery, and access to plentiful food is not the daily challenge it is in many other countries.

God knows that our current focus on material goods will not make us happy. While our consumption of goods skyrockets, the number of teen suicides rises. Divorce rates have stabilized at the highest rate in history. More people are depressed. Rates of stress-related illnesses, such as heart disease and stroke, are soaring.

God never suggests that happiness should be our goal in life, but rather our purpose should be enjoying a relationship with Him and glorifying Him with our lives. The Lord declares this through Jeremiah:

Let not the wise man boast of his wisdom
  or the strong man boast of his strength
  or the rich man boast of his riches,
but let him who boasts boast about this:
  that he understands and knows me,
that I am the Lord who exercises kindness,
  justice, and righteousness on earth" (Jeremiah 9:23–24).

Instead, we seek the easy answer rather than the best one. God wants us to face our problems, including illness, from His perspective and find joy in trusting Him. As often as necessary, He will bring us back to frustration with the world's answers until we learn to value only the contentment found in knowing Him deeply. God wants us to understand that only our relationship with Him will lead to real contentment, a state much more valuable and lasting than the happiness the world offers.

I Am King of the World

We don't always get what we want, the Rolling Stones sing in a popular song, but sometimes when we try, we do get what we need. This is especially true for believers in God's grace and providence. When we know and begin to follow God, we can trust that anything that happens in our lives is at the very least allowed by Him—if not planned by Him—for our ultimate good. We often don't realize this at the time. However, I know that some of the "worst" things that have happened in my life turned out to be much better for me in the long run than the alternatives I would have chosen had not God blocked my path.

For example, when I learned that I had lung cancer I was extremely anxious to have the cancer removed but had to wait over a month for the surgery. During that time my surgeon was developing a new system for pain relief that would deliver painkillers directly to a surgical site. With our permission, he tested this on me. The lung removal was the most painful of all my surgeries, and I cannot imagine undergoing it without this new technology. Had I been allowed to choose the date of my surgery (and I would have chosen to have it immediately), the pain would have been much worse.

Christians recognize the truth of one God who rules over this world and the next. Unfortunately, believers in this one true God often act as if they, rather than God, are almighty and all-knowing. When we relinquish this myth, we grow strong in our faith and able to witness with our lives, being yielded to God's will with true peace and joy.

If God is almighty, omniscient, and loving, as we know He is, then He controls and knows about everything. When we worry and work at making something happen, we simply affirm our lack of faith that God is who He is. Often I start my prayer time with an urgent request of God, something that I think needs His attention. After patiently explaining this to Him, I begin to realize how ridiculous my petition is. God already knows the situation, already loves the people involved, and already exists in tomorrow. What I need to do is thank Him for His love and pray that everyone involved will come to know Him better, love Him more, and trust Him completely. Then I should ask forgiveness for not acknowledging these things with my every breath.

Oswald Chambers, author of *My Utmost for His Highest,* the most widely read devotional of all time, reminds us:

> The initiative of the saint is not toward self-realization, but towards knowing Jesus Christ. The spiritual saint never believes circumstances to be haphazard, or thinks of his life as secular and sacred; *he sees everything he is dumped down in as the means of securing the knowledge of Jesus Christ...* Self-realization leads to the enthronement of work whereas the saint enthrones Jesus Christ in his work... The aim of the spiritual saint is "that I may know Him" (emphasis added).

Every morning, after I thank God for the day and ask Him to make me a blessing, I also ask Him to keep my face turned toward His light. When I do this, I affirm that He is almighty; His love will light my path if I allow it to. When I try to substitute my own puny knowledge and might, anxiety and failure follow.

We must resolve repeatedly to trust in His love for us, against our nature and against Satan's attempts to make us fearful and keep us busy fixing ourselves. On the night I finally realized the futility of trying to control my own life, I was awake working on a difficult problem and praying for *God's help* in coming up with *my* answer.

I was amazed when God answered my prayer by assuring me of His love and power and telling me to leave it to Him. I had always felt self-reliant and had been sure that I would be able to find an answer this time also. But after hours of agonizing, I finally prayed, "Lord, I still don't know what to do or what will happen. But from now on I am going to trust that you love me more than I can imagine and you are taking care of me because of that love. No matter what my outward circumstances are, I will believe that you are in them and follow you." God gave me a sense of assurance that has never left me and has made all the difference after I prayed what Catherine Marshall calls, in *Beyond Ourselves,* a "prayer of relinquishment." I believe that on that night Jesus Christ entered into my life at a deeper level than I had previously allowed Him, and He began to teach me what it meant for Him to be both my Lord and my Savior. I am thankful that I will have time to be eternally grateful to Him for this!

A Classic Answer to Prayer

Many of us have agonized about some situation and realized later that God had control of it all the time. St. Augustine's mother, Monica, provides the classic example. Monica prayed unceasingly for her son, a wayward young man involved in all the sins of the world that mothers fear. He had determined to leave his mother and his hometown of Alexandria and go to Rome.

Monica knew he would face even more temptations in Rome and prayed the entire night before his ship was to sail that he would be prevented from leaving. Her prayer seemed reasonable, but God did not answer as she wanted. It was a good thing for the rest of us that Augustine did go to Rome, where he met Saint Ambrose, was converted, and became one of the greatest thinkers in Christian church history.

Lessons from Scripture

When I forget this lesson, I turn to Scripture to remind me. Psalms are especially helpful here, because they include the entire story: fear, anger, discouragement, frustration, confusion, and peace. As do many other people, I find Psalm 23 comforting: "The Lord is my shepherd: I shall not be in want." Notice that David does not say, "I usually have what I need." God promises that we can follow our shepherd with no anxiety.

But the Psalms are not all completely peaceful. In Asaph's Psalm 73 we see the progression of the psalmist through various phases before he reaches the same conclusion as David. Asaph is frustrated by the "prosperity of the wicked," who "have no struggles" (vv. 3–4). We have all been where Asaph is. In contrast to the wicked, whose arrogance makes us angry, we have been plagued all day long. We wonder why we must deal with illness, deceit, money troubles, or betrayal. Finally, however, in a wonderful crescendo of praise and peace, Asaph proclaims:

> My flesh and my heart may fail,
>   but God is the strength of my heart
>   and my portion forever...
>
> I have made the Sovereign Lord my refuge;
>   I will tell of all your deeds (vv. 26–28).

I am grateful that God has taught me that He knows and I do not. He understands that we will forget to trust Him. He desires that we will do this less as we grow in our walk with Him.

Me First

Unfortunately, in the good times we have a tendency to return to worshiping ourselves. When my days are sunny, I may forget to pick up my Bible. I seem to be doing well at controlling my own life. I pray, yet I feel no compulsion to connect further with God. But when I am sick, a family problem looms, or I don't have an answer for a difficult question, I run to Scripture and seek God's grace in prayer. God wants to teach us that He must be first in our lives.

In the Lord's Prayer, Jesus teaches us to ask God, "Give us this day our daily bread." Another time He reminds us that man does not live by bread alone and that true life requires more than physical bread. We receive this "bread" by putting God first in our lives in terms of time and energy commitment. As long as we think more about our struggles, our illness, and our daily difficulties than we do about God, we will not grow in ways that will provide us with real bread.

As we learn to love God, we naturally begin to work at loving others better. Realizing what we have been given leads us to share it with others rather than focusing on ourselves. In his play *Our Town*, Thornton Wilder presents the ghost of a young woman who has died in childbirth and is allowed to go back to see her life. She talks with the Stage Manager (a character who provides the narration for the play) and another dead person, Simon Stimson, about living through her sixteenth birthday for the second time:

> **Emily:** It goes so fast. We don't have time to look at one another... I didn't realize. So all that was going on and we never noticed... Do any human beings ever realize life while they live it?—every, every minute?
>
> **Stage Manager:** No... The saints and poets, maybe—they do some.
>
> **Emily:** I should have listened to you. That's all human beings are! Just blind people!
>
> **Simon Stimson:** Yes, now you know. That's what it was to be alive. To move about in a cloud of ignorance; to

go up and down trampling on the feelings of those about you. To spend and waste time as though you had a million years. To be always at the mercy of one self-centered passion or another.

We search for happiness through fame, fortune, serial relationships, and acclaim. Yet daily we read reports of the suicides of rich people, the painful ending of yet another celebrity marriage, or the downward spiral of someone who was once at the top of whatever game he or she played. The "saints and poets" Wilder writes about have the opportunity to "realize life" because they see their lives through God's eyes. God clearly teaches us that "me first" always leads to despair, and the only important thing we do with our lives on earth is to love God and others.

Loving others also distracts us from our own pain and difficulty. When I was pregnant with Carey, Rick and I attended a Lamaze childbirth class where we practiced breathing exercises designed to aid in coping with the pain of labor and delivery. The instructor directed the prospective mothers to concentrate on something across the room and breathe as we had been taught. At the same time, our partners squeezed our thighs, and none of us felt much pain. Then she had our partners squeeze again while we were not breathing and concentrating, and we all yelped.

This exercise showed us the power of thinking about something other than what was going on in our bodies. I used Lamaze breathing and focused concentration through twenty-four hours of labor and many other times when recuperating from surgeries or undergoing painful tests such as the needle biopsy of my lung. I know firsthand the power of concentrating on something other than myself!

God wants us to put Him first because He knows that is best for us. His plan includes concentrating on Him and loving others as a natural outgrowth of knowing Him. As usual, His plan leads to greater pleasure and less pain for us than our plans ever will.

Chasing after the Wind

Recently, Rick and I visited a local retirement community to begin future planning and were pleasantly surprised by the facilities and wonderful programs available. We talked about the good things we could look forward to there.

When we came home and looked at the financial information the retirement community representatives had given us, we began to worry. Were we saving enough money to afford to move there? Could we be happy in a smaller, less comfortable place? Should we buy long-term care insurance? What would happen if one of us needed nursing care for an extended time? We had been hooked into a trap: worrying about our physical future on earth.

As human beings, we are naturally concerned about our daily lives, but here on earth we are only at the beginning of our life's journey. As believers in the one true God, we must gain an eternal perspective in a world that emphasizes passing pleasures and disposable relationships. We cannot imagine the future, including the afterlife, but we can believe that *God is already there.* Obviously that means that whatever comes, we are covered. This does not mean that we will not experience pain and heartbreak; we will. God chooses not to eliminate these from our lives. But we can trust that God is taking care of this world in better ways than we could and that we will enjoy eternity with Him in ways we cannot conceive of.

Why doesn't God just let us know what the future holds and what heaven will be like? The answer is twofold. First, since we agree that God loves us, we can assume that we are better off not knowing. If it were loving to tell us about the future, you can be sure He would. Earthly life is a training ground for trusting God, and uncertainty is necessary for this training to be complete. After all, we can't trust something if we are certain it will or will not happen.

Second, we have amazing abilities to think and reason, but we are not in the same league with God. Because of this we need to learn to live with mystery. The great English novelist Anthony Trollope even went so far as to say, "Without God there is no mystery."

Let me explain by using an incident with our dog, Dante, who has been an important part of our family for fourteen years. The other day Dante rested in the doorway, as usual, while Rick and I were doing the dishes together and kidding with each other using lines from the long-running off-Broadway musical *The Fantasticks*.

Rick said, "This plum is too ripe!" to which I replied loudly, "Sorry!" Dante's ears pricked up.

"You were about to drown that magnolia!" Rick continued. I shouted back, "Sorry!" At this point, Dante became agitated because he was not used to raised voices between us. He got up, came over to us, and barked.

I explained to him that everything was fine; we were just pretending to be actors playing the roles of the grumpy fathers in *The Fantasticks*. Dante, of course, understood nothing of this. However, my tone of voice was reassuring. Furthermore, since he has a long-term relationship with me that has taught him he can trust me, his concern evaporated, and he soon went back to sleep.

Dante's reaction reminds me of our desire to know God's plans. A dog could never understand actors and plays. We could never understand completely who God is and what His actions mean here on earth. The dog may be momentarily upset, but when he remembers our relationship and hears our comforting voices, he calms down. He assumes that we know more than he does and goes along for the ride, expecting and receiving the love and attention he needs when he asks for it. This is just what we should be doing daily in our relationship with God.

Solomon, the writer of Ecclesiastes, reminds us, "He has also set eternity in the hearts of men; yet they cannot fathom what God has done from beginning to end... As for men, God tests them so that they may see that they are like the animals" (Ecclesiastes 3:11, 18). What a good realization to incorporate into our daily lives! When we believe in our deepest heart that God's mysterious purposes will ultimately be worked out for our good, our anxiety disappears, our blood pressure lowers, and we are healthier. Learning to live with the mystery of God allows our bodies the rest they need to face their daily challenges.

What We Can Do to Change Our Life Attitudes

Being sick is not fun. I continue to pray for healing of my body while I am here on earth. But I have learned ways to cope with the body God has given me today. Rather than insisting that I cannot be happy unless I am cured of my illness, I give thanks for all the blessings God is showering on me today, especially those I don't usually notice.

Give It Up

Growing older even without a major illness often involves a series of "giving up" stages: giving up work, giving up the family home, giving up driving. Chronic illness often forces us to give up many activities we loved before the illness.

For instance, I used to enjoy knitting. Although I never measured it, I am sure that my blood pressure naturally lowered when I knit. But I can no longer use this natural relaxation treatment because my fingers, wrists, and elbows are too crooked and sore. Occasionally I will buy some yarn on sale, thinking that perhaps I could knit a few minutes per day. But I pay for these experiments with several days of splints, icing, and aspirin cream. I have learned that I *can crochet* for a few minutes at a time, which substitutes when I am really needlework-deprived. I can also embroider occasionally, a hobby that I had not done for years.

I also used to love gardening; digging in the dirt always worked for me as a sure cure for the blahs. Now I cannot plant, weed, or mulch. For two years friends and paid helpers have tended my garden, hoping that I will be able to play in it again. This past year I tore out my rosebushes in order to make the garden less difficult to manage. I am beginning to think about the delights of window boxes.

Step 1 in the process of changing your attitude is accepting the limitations that disease has put on your body. For instance, I know that I will not knit again. I know that I can't play the piano for hours anymore. I cannot sail or row a boat. Because we have a ladder into the lake, I can swim, but not very far. I can't have a marathon Christmas cookie-baking day. I cannot travel to New York City to visit my daughter. I am not able to help my son move into his new apartment. I don't like these limits, but once I accept that they are real, I can grieve them and move on in my life.

Embrace Our Limitations

Now comes the good part. I make a list of the things I can still do with the gifts that God has given me and continues to give me every day. I can crochet. I can play some piano. I can usually still get into and out of a rowboat so that Rick can row me around the lake. I can bake a few Christmas cookies (probably still more than we really need). We have the financial resources to help Carey come home to visit from the Big Apple. Although I cannot clean Mark's apartment, I can make curtains for him on my own schedule.

John 1:16 reminds us, "From the fullness of his grace we have all received one blessing after another." When I remember this, I can embrace change as one of God's blessings. This year I have finally realized that I am no longer a gardener; I used to be a gardener. It is alright that I no longer garden. In fact, when the garden gets out of control completely or it becomes too expensive for someone else to tend it, we are thinking of having a "closing the garden" party, where we invite our friends to bring pots and shovels and take our garden away to their houses. Sounds like fun to me. I can buy four or five of the most exotic, expensive plants I want and create one amazing window box.

Choose Joy

My eighty-eight-year-old friend Ethel has lovingly cared for her husband Joe through years of dementia. In a recent conversation Ethel told me about a research project she had begun. She has bought a notebook in which she writes every use of the word *joy* she finds in the media, Scripture, and other reading. Ethel then writes a commentary on the meaning of joy in the context where she finds it. She wants to know what joy really is and has concluded that what we are being told in today's media does not coincide with what Scripture teaches. For example, a Christian will never find joy in the latest video games, serial relationships, or carefree vacations. I am in awe of Ethel's commitment to lifelong learning, to caring for Joe, and to choosing joy in such a difficult situation. Her choices inspire me and others in her life.

When I am thinking clearly from God's perspective, I find that I have much more to be thankful for than I have to complain about: a wonderful family, amazing friends, a strong faith, a loving and faithful God, a country in which I am free to do almost anything I choose, the sun in the morning, and the moon at night. When I find myself complaining about something,

I am embarrassed. As Francis Schaeffer said, "When I am in the presence of God, it seems profoundly unbecoming to demand anything."

Almost everything in my life can be seen as burden or blessing. For example, I have three shelves in one closet completely full with several months' supply of medicines and supplements. This could be seen as a symbol of my being trapped in my illness or as a display of the blessings of modern medicine; doctors today are able to treat illnesses that were virtually untreatable even fifty years ago. I spend over an hour a day doing various exercises, which could be seen as a waste of my time or as a wonderful alternative to being in a wheelchair. The ring splints on my fingers help to keep my joints from curving so badly that I cannot use them. When young women ask me where I got those "cool rings" and I tell them they are available by prescription at the hospital, I realize the rings, too, are a blessing. I would like to be free of medicines and their side effects, not need to exercise in order to be able to move, and have my hands look good and work well. But I do not let Satan steal my joy by prompting me to focus on my limitations rather than my blessings.

The secular world recently tapped into the idea of counting your blessings. The *Journal of Personality and Social Psychology* reports that participants in a three-week study slept longer, felt more refreshed, and were happier with their lives when they wrote a daily list naming five things they were grateful for. Science apparently affirms that we are more satisfied when we realize that we are blessed. The popular media headlined this study for several months, showing we are eager for good news.

As long as we complain about our limitations and focus on our losses, we sap the energy God gave us to use today. He always has blessings in mind for us, but we must stop saying no to them before He can bestow them fully. Maybe we also need to see the blessings that are already there. I urge you to make this a matter of continuing prayer, since you will be tempted every day to give in to feeling sorry for yourself rather than recognizing that you are enormously blessed.

Enjoy the Seasons of Life

Rick and I were married during our senior year of college, and we both worked several jobs to make ends meet. As a part-time bus driver, Rick called the bus coordinator at the garage every morning between 7:30 and 8:00 and said, "Ray, this is Wallace. What do you have for me today?" We would be pleased if there was a route for him to take, and Ray would tell him where and when he would be working.

I often think of Rick's checking in with Ray as an illustration for my relationship with God. When I am paying attention to this relationship, I check in with Him every morning, ask "What do you have for me today?" and then do my best to fulfill the assignment. My job has nothing to do with that day's physical challenges. God knows all about them, and His assignments are always commensurate with my abilities. He may sometimes stretch us beyond our comfort zones, but He will never ask the impossible of us, no matter what season we are living through.

Living through Seasons

Every climate on earth has seasons. Even countries with continuous tropical temperatures have rainy and dry seasons. Humans begin as babies and, if we are blessed with many years on earth, end as old people. Living with chronic illness can help us to embrace the seasons in our lives more joyfully.

As a young wife and mother in the late 1960s and early 1970s, I was taught that women could have it all, juggling a full-time career and home with aplomb. Fortunately the Lord managed to teach me that this was unrealistic for me before I died trying to prove that I was superwoman. But the fact that I had my first heart attack at age forty-seven is probably related to the fact that I stressed my body and soul by working too much at the things of this world.

Now I see that people can have it all, but not all at the same time. When my children were babies and toddlers, during my spring season, I worked part time at my private counseling practice. This allowed me to do the work that God had gifted me to do and that I loved, added to our household income, and allowed me some hours of talking with adults. Rick and I arranged our schedules so that he was usually available to care for the kids while I worked, and vice versa.

As Carey and Mark got older, my summer time, I worked more in my practice and taught at several colleges and universities. Because of my flexible schedule I continued to be active in their lives, even homeschooling them for several years. I love being a mother and am grateful that God allowed me health when my kids were young so that I could play games, walk, bake, make crafts, and play music with them. I loved creating things with Carey and accompanying Mark's violin-playing on the piano.

I am now in my autumn years. Many of these things I can no longer do; some I can do in a limited way. Last Christmas, for instance, Mark and I got out some of his old music and played together. I also taught my family how to make the special German Christmas cookie my grandmother used to bake. Our Christmas celebration actually seems more blessed because we are less busy with physically demanding tasks.

Seasons as Part of God's Plan

I believe that God gives us seasons in part to prepare us for changes our bodies encounter as we age, perhaps sooner with chronic illness. I know that my winter will come early, unless my life ends suddenly while I am still enjoying autumn. I hope to embrace the next season joyfully and make the most of every day God grants me. He has a purpose for every breath I take, and I must spend my energy finding it and fulfilling it.

My much younger friend, Marilyn, found herself with time on her hands when her daughter left for college and her husband accepted a mission opportunity that required him to be away from home a lot. Instead of feeling sorry for herself or complaining, Marilyn told me she had "decided to follow the example of Dorcas" by making clothes for the poor in her spare time like Dorcas did in Acts 9. Marilyn follows her family tradition in being a skilled seamstress and needle worker. But now, as well as adorning herself and her family with these skills, she spends hours finishing off unused yarn and cloth making clothing and quilts for her church's thrift store. She donates her gifts and time to those who need them and knows that her creations are truly appreciated. I receive an added benefit from Marilyn's decision; I now have a place to donate the yarn and fabric I can no longer work with myself!

We can make Marilyn's choice. Every day we should honor God by embracing the self He has created for this season in our life and deciding to love Him through it.

Lighten Your Load for the Journey

My parents had lived in their home for thirty-five years when they decided to move to a retirement community. I knew from experience that moving would take a lot of energy, but I was really not prepared for sorting through every material belonging they had accumulated in their sixty years together. The amount of furniture, clothing, kitchen utensils, tools, toys, books, and decorations daunted us. But going through high school Latin projects, eighth-grade diplomas, moth-eaten but special embroidered pillowcases, cookbooks, and boxes of photographs (identified and unidentified) proved overwhelming. Each of these objects required an explanation, a weighing of options, a decision. Almost every other day for weeks my mother and I sorted and packed.

Moving my parents' things prompted me to begin this process in my own life. Although I learned a lot about their lives through packing for the move, I wished that Mom and Dad had done some of this earlier when they were still able to discern what was important to pass on and to share stories with their grandchildren about the objects they thought worthy of keeping.

Jesus tells us clearly that our earthly possessions can reflect our vanity. For example, in Luke 12 He tells the story of the rich man who decides to build new barns for his grain and goods and then dies that night. Jesus' conclusion is that the full scope of a person's existence does not consist in an abundance of possessions. One Christian author suggests that we should think of everything we own as having a sign on it that states, "Soon to be burned."

When my siblings and I cleaned out my parents' apartment after my mother's death, we each took carloads of things to our homes and made several trips to the Salvation Army. But we said goodbye to each other in a driveway filled with things designated for trash pickup. Seeing our parents' possessions passed out among children and grandchildren, sent to charity, or thrown out should underline this message for us: what lasts is our relationship with God and how we love others because of that relationship. Everything else is "chasing after the wind" as the writer of Ecclesiastes reminds us.

Beginning the Process

This fall I went through my jewelry box and sorted out the things I never wear or that have no significance to me. When Carey came home to visit, I offered her first choice of any of these things before they went to the local charity store. Then we went through what I had kept, and I explained who had given me what and on what occasion, which pieces were heirlooms and whom they had belonged to, and why certain jewelry had special meaning. We even labeled things for future reference. Now I can easily find the jewelry I really do wear, and I know that Carey understands what she will one day inherit and choose for herself what she wants to keep.

I don't smoke, drink, or gamble, but I love to buy books, a vice I inherited from my parents and passed on to my children. (Carey recently told us that when she was young she thought there were two kinds of money: regular money, to be used for most things, was limited, but money for books was unlimited.) When my mother died, the thought of integrating her books into our household prompted me to begin culling our book collection down to two large bookcases. Although I still have cutting to do, I have given away hundreds of books in the past two years, and already I can more easily find books to read or lend to a friend. The thought of being able to move into a retirement home without storing boxes of books somewhere spurs me on.

How and Why to Choose

Take a good long look at your stuff. You will probably find that most of it does not add to your satisfaction in life. Our stuff often weighs us down so that we cannot concentrate on the important things—our relationships with God and others. Owning things requires taking care of them, finding places to store them, worrying about them, insuring them, and arranging to pass them down to others.

At the same time, some people throw things out indiscriminately, leaving no physical mementoes for their children or other relatives. Rather than going to this extreme, choose what is special to you and worth saving. When my grandparents sold their house, I lived hundreds of miles away. My parents offered to send me anything I would like from their home, and

I asked for a small glass paperweight. I remembered vividly sitting on my grandmother's scratchy horsehair sofa looking at its multicolored glass flowers. Even today looking at that paperweight summons the smells of my grandparents' house: Bapa's cigars, Grammie's roasts, old books. Having physical reminders of our forefathers and foremothers gives us a sense of being grounded in a family—something larger than ourselves.

Your precious things will make more sense to others if you choose them now and explain their significance to those who love you. Carey and Mark know why the small paperweight is displayed in our living room. When I am gone they can decide whether or not they want to continue to honor that particular memento or give it to someone else who will enjoy it, either in the family or outside.

Getting down to a more basic lifestyle in which you own only those things you actually use or which are very precious to you is remarkably freeing. Physical baggage often leads us to focus on our past in a vain effort to hang onto it. Do I really need my class notes from college? Must I have copies of my elementary school report cards? How about keeping the paint-by-number picture I made sixty years ago that was ugly then and ugly and old now? Giving away or throwing out such things frees energy to focus on the here and now.

In addition, being free of stuff from the past will make my living space today easier to navigate. Baking has always been one of my passions, and over the years I accumulated a vast collection of utensils. Recently I found I was having trouble being able to find and reach what I wanted from my cupboards. I packed up gadgets I hadn't used in years and put them in a box in the basement. When I was sure I wouldn't want them again, I donated the box. Rick helped me re-arrange the things I actually use in my baking so that I access them without the trouble and pain I had been having. And he gets more cookies!

If the task of cleaning out your life seems too daunting, try asking a friend to help you. You can always disagree with your friend and keep whatever you think is indispensable. But you will have a more objective person to help you unload the unnecessary, and you can share memories along the way.

Learn to Empathize

I remember being a passenger when my mother was looking for a parking place in a lot. Another woman pulled into a handicap parking place, got out, and walked into the store. My mother commented, "Her handicap must be mental!" I thought my mom's quip was hilarious at the time. Now I recognize that we had no idea what that woman might have been dealing with on a day-to-day basis.

I now have a handicap tag for my car. Often I use it on days when I am not walking well. Sometimes I simply have very little energy. Occasionally my lungs are giving me trouble. None of these things show on the outside of my body, and I sometimes wonder if people question why I am parking in a handicap slot.

Being ill has taught me to empathize. I remember distinctly when I looked down on a woman who wore orthopedic shoes like those I wear every day. Now I am grateful that such shoes exist, because they drastically reduce my danger of falling and alleviate my back pain. But when I was young, I thought women should always dress fashionably, no matter what the cost to their personal comfort.

When I am well enough, friends and neighbors see me doing things like getting mail from the mailbox, walking down the street, or shopping. Most of them never realize that many days I cannot reach the mailbox or get into a car or even walk to the corner. When I answer the phone, people often say, "You sound great!" On the rare occasion that I go to a family party, I prepare for it by resting for hours or even days so that I can be there and leave when my "battery dies." I may spend days resting afterward, but family members usually are completely unaware of this. To hide my weaknesses and avoid talking about painful topics, I usually don't share how I am feeling, thus feeding into the myth that everything is all right.

When I talk with others who live with chronic illness, I learn that this is normal for most of us, so I can reliably trust that many people I see "functioning" in the world are really not doing all that well either. They may even need an extra hand or an especially bright smile. The grumpy woman ahead of us in line may be in pain. The man who cuts in front of us at the gas station may be hurrying to see his child in the hospital. The obnoxious child at the movie theater may be grieving that his parent has cancer.

Even if people are not struggling with an illness, they are probably struggling in some way. The older I get the more I realize that most of us really have no idea what others are going through most of the time. As God's followers we should admit this and try to remedy it.

Value Your Own Contributions

One of the brightest university students I ever had the privilege to teach is confined to a wheelchair by multiple sclerosis. He told me about going on a date to a restaurant where the waitress asked his girlfriend what he would like to eat. The waitress assumed that because he was unable to walk, he was also unable to read a menu, choose a meal, and speak for himself. In relating this humiliating experience to me, he echoed the famous line of the disability movement: "How should you treat a person with a disability? Like a person."

Our society values success. When we are not "successful" in our health, others may minimize us as human beings.

However, we do not have to let others' definitions become our definition. The fact that they do not understand or respect our situation should remain their problem. Remember the famous words of Eleanor Roosevelt: "No one can make you feel inferior without your consent."

If we are in a wheelchair, confined to home, or walking freely about but unable to function for more than a few hours at a time, we can still be contributing to the world by filling God's purpose for our days. That is the only yardstick I use in measuring myself. When I take a long look at other measures, they all fall short of the mark.

Doing Well from God's Perspective

My friend Carol, whom I wrote about in chapter 6, had a problem with her heartbeat. The procedure her surgeon performed not only did not solve the problem but also left her with a pacemaker for life. After changing cardiologists and surgeons, Carol scheduled another surgery to stop some erratic heartbeats (ventricular tachycardia, or VT) that caused her to be lightheaded and contributed to the possibility of her having a heart attack.

In years of dealing with chronic heart failure, Carol has learned to trust in God's guidance, and her spiritual life has deepened. I have watched her grow more joyful even as her body gives her more difficulty. Praise is always on her lips, as the psalmist states (34:1).

Carol had to wait for the procedure, but she did not fret. Her previous experiences led to recurring fears of a bad outcome, but most of the time Carol understood deeply that God was in control. While she was praying several weeks before her surgery date, Carol felt prompted to ask God to cure her erratic heartbeat. Immediately she felt a sense of well-being and felt God had healed her. She never consciously experienced another VT episode.

When the surgery date arrived, the surgeon was unable to make her heart misbehave by going into VT, which was the first step in "fixing" the problem. After several attempts, he labeled the procedure unsuccessful and abandoned the surgery. We thought that Carol would have to learn to live with the aberrant heartbeats. Later, when Carol was speaking by phone to her cardiologist's nurse, she asked the nurse to check the data from her heart monitor to see when her last VT occurred. The nurse hesitated to check all the data until Carol explained to her that she thought she had an answer to prayer. Some minutes passed before the nurse returned with the answer: the last problem heartbeat happened six weeks earlier, three weeks before her procedure, exactly the day she had prayed for healing.

I delight in the fact that Carol's heart was healed. But the important fact to remember is that Carol's healing came about *after* she had learned to trust God with the future, no matter what it held, and to praise Him every day for His blessings. Carol's faith would not have been lessened if her heartbeat had remained erratic. Perhaps the most important change God desires in our life attitude is for us to demonstrate this kind of trust in His love for us.

Does this mean that we should pray for miraculous physical healing of our illnesses and be disappointed if they do not occur? None of us knows why some physical healings occur as a result of prayer and some do not. Richard Dominguez addresses this question scripturally in his book *Caring for Your Wife in Sickness and in Health*:

> The major thing I notice in these verses [James 5:14–16] is that nowhere does it say that the sick person will be miraculously healed or even that the sick person will always be healed; it doesn't even say that we will be healed in this life. What it does say is that we are to pray

over a believer who is sick... I believe we can pray for miracles and expect them to happen. [However] ... if it is miraculous, it is equally unpredictable. We are to seek the Lord's will, but we can never forget that it is *His* will, not ours.

Very few of us will experience a dramatic example of physical healing in our lifetimes. But all believers have already experienced spiritual healing through the life, death, and resurrection of Jesus Christ and can look forward to eternity spent in God's presence. In a very real sense, we have been "healed" of everything worth being healed of. Our lives should abound in gratitude and joy for this amazing gift, no matter what battles our bodies face on a daily basis.

Most of us would not choose to live with a chronic illness. Sickness brings pain to our families, our friends, and us. Being ill costs time, money, and energy, disrupts our plans, and causes us to question everything. But we have opportunities with these trials. We learn to be more in tune with our bodies and respect what they do for us. We have the opportunity to be more aware of and responsive to the unspoken needs of others. Our friends become even dearer to us. If we allow it, we grow closer to God, driven to Him in times of difficulty. We gain an eternal perspective on life. We learn to praise instead of complain. We glorify God, and He comforts and encourages us. Praise Him, for His mercy endures forever!

In Summary

1. God intends contentment for us, not happiness.
2. Everything in our life is either allowed or planned by God.
3. Our "me first" attitudes lead to despair.
4. We can trust God even though the future is a mystery.

5. To change our life attitudes, we must consistently thank Him for all the blessings He showers on us.

6. God gives us seasons of life, and if we adjust to change rather than complain, our contentment grows.

7. The things God gives to us can sometimes make us happier when we give them to someone else.

8. Being ill can teach us how to love and accept the behavior of others and to value our own unique contributions to this world.

10. God has given us the gift of salvation and eternal life with Him, which encourages us to trust and praise Him, no matter what is happening in our physical bodies.

Chapter Ten

Strength for Today
and Bright Hope for Tomorrow

You will learn:

- to seek God's grace through prayer and Scripture

Your word is a lamp to my feet
and a light for my path.

PSALM 119:105

*A*ll of the principles we have discussed thus far are true and helpful in dealing with illness. However, in the midst of great pain, when you are exhausted, when trials come at you in groups rather than singly, in situations that seem to be veering completely out of control, you can forget great principles and sink into despair. As I mentioned in chapter 6, these are times when you should seek God's grace even more through prayer and Scripture.

But when you are depressed, you may not feel like even opening your Bible. For such times, I keep a small notebook filled with verses and quotations that, in my best times, I have chosen to read in my worst times. Most are Bible verses, but some of the quotations are from Christians and others who have experienced pain and difficulty and found solace in God's love.

I suggest that you begin to collect such tidbits for yourself to be used when you need them most. Here are some of my favorites to get you started.

~

Rejoice in the Lord always. I will say it again: Rejoice! . . . The Lord is near. Do not be anxious about anything, but in everything, by prayer and petition, with thanksgiving, present your requests to God. And the peace of God, which transcends all understanding, will guard your hearts and your minds in Christ Jesus.

—Philippians 4:4–7

The Lord your God is with you,
he is mighty to save.
He will take great delight in you,
he will quiet you with his love,
he will rejoice over you with singing.

—Zephaniah 3:17

The God of all grace... will himself restore you and make you strong, firm and steadfast.

—1 PETER 5:10

The Lord is my strength and my shield;
    my heart trusts in him, and I am helped.
My heart leaps for joy
    and I will give thanks to him in song.

—PSALM 28:7

And we know that in all things God works for the good of those who love him, who have been called according to his purpose.

—ROMANS 8:28

God is our refuge and strength,
    an ever-present help in trouble.

—PSALM 46:1

He heals the brokenhearted
    and binds up their wounds.

—PSALM 147:3

Cast your cares on the Lord
    and he will sustain you.

—PSALM 55:22

I have... covered you with the shadow of my hand.

—ISAIAH 51:16

The Lord is my light and my salvation.

—PSALM 27:1

Fretting springs from a determination to get our own way. Our Lord never worried and He was never anxious, because He was not out to realize His own ideas; He was out to realize God's ideas.

—OSWALD CHAMBERS, *MY UTMOST FOR HIS HIGHEST*

Do not fear, for I am with you;
    do not be dismayed, for I am your God.
I will strengthen you and help you;
    I will uphold you with my righteous right hand.

—ISAIAH 41:10

I will say of the Lord, "He is my refuge and my fortress,
    my God, in whom I trust."

—PSALM 91:2

Heal me, O Lord, and I will be healed;
    save me and I will be saved,
    for you are the one I praise.

—JEREMIAH 17:14

My flesh and my heart may fail,
    but God is the strength of my heart
    and my portion forever.

—PSALM 73:26

For men are not cast off
    by the Lord forever.
Though he brings grief, he will show compassion,
    so great is his unfailing love.
For he does not willingly bring affliction
    or grief to the children of men.

—LAMENTATIONS 3:31–33

In this world you will have trouble. But take heart! I have over-
come the world.

—John 16:33

> The Lord is good,
>> a refuge in times of trouble.
> He cares for those who trust in him.

—Nahum 1:7

Finally, brothers, whatever is true, whatever is noble, whatever is
right, whatever is pure, whatever is lovely, whatever is admirable—
if anything is excellent or praiseworthy—think about such things.

—Philippians 4:8

He has delivered us from such a deadly peril, and he will deliver
us. On him we have set our hope that he will continue to deliver
us, as you help us by your prayers. Then many will give thanks
on our behalf for the gracious favor granted us in answer to the
prayers of many.

—2 Corinthians 1:10–11

I know what it is to be in need, and I know what it is to have
plenty. I have learned the secret of being content in any and every
situation, whether well fed or hungry, whether living in plenty or
in want. I can do everything through him who gives me strength.

—Philippians 4:12–13

> When I am afraid,
>> I will trust in you.
> In God, whose word I praise,
>> in God I trust; I will not be afraid.
> What can mortal man do to me?

—Psalm 56:3–4

Open my eyes that I may see
    wonderful things in your law.

—P<small>SALM</small> 119:18

I call on the Lord in my distress,
    and he answers me.

—P<small>SALM</small> 120:1

My help comes from the Lord,
    the Maker of heaven and earth...
he who watches over you will not... slumber nor sleep...
the Lord will watch over your coming and going
    both now and forevermore.

—P<small>SALM</small> 121:2–4, 8

Those who trust in the Lord are like Mount Zion,
which cannot be shaken but endures forever.

—P<small>SALM</small> 125:1

I know that you can do all things;
    no plan of yours can be thwarted.

—J<small>OB</small> 42:2

The joy of the Lord is [my] strength.

—N<small>EHEMIAH</small> 8:10

We rejoice that He is on the throne and knows us by name.

—C<small>ARL</small> F. H. H<small>ENRY</small>

If God has let you suffer, it is because He sees something good
in it.
    Trust Him.

—P<small>OPE</small> J<small>OHN</small> P<small>AUL</small> II

But I trust in you, O Lord;
    I say, "You are my God."
My times are in your hands.

              —PSALM 31:14–15

The Lord will guide you always.

              —ISAIAH 58:11

Trust in the Lord with all your heart
    and lean not on your own understanding;
in all your ways acknowledge him,
    and he will make your paths straight.

              —PROVERBS 3:5–6

I sought the Lord, and he answered me;
    he delivered me from all my fears.
Those who look to him are radiant;
    their faces are never covered with shame.

              —PSALM 34:4–5

A righteous man may have many troubles,
    but the Lord delivers him from them all.

              —PSALM 34:19

Cast all your anxiety on him because he cares for you.

              —1 PETER 5:7

Your beauty should not come from outward adornment, such as braided hair and the wearing of gold jewelry and fine clothes. Instead, it should be that of your inner self, the unfading beauty of a gentle and quiet spirit, which is of great worth in God's sight.

              —1 PETER 3:4

The Lord's unfailing love
  surrounds the man who trusts in him.

—Psalm 32:10

You intended to harm me, but God intended it for good to accomplish what is now being done, the saving of many lives. So then, don't be afraid.

—Genesis 50:20–21

My eyes are ever on the Lord,
  for only he will release my feet from the snare.

—Psalm 25:15

Some trust in chariots and some in horses,
  but we trust in the name of the Lord our God.

—Psalm 20:7

Great peace have they who love your law,
  and nothing can make them stumble.

—Psalm 119:165

I waited patiently for the Lord;
  he turned to me and heard my cry.
He lifted me out of the slimy pit,
  out of the mud and mire;
he set my feet on a rock
  and gave me a firm place to stand.
He put a new song in my mouth,
  a hymn of praise to our God.
Many will see and fear
  and put their trust in the Lord.

—Psalm 40:1–3

Create in me a pure heart, O God,
    and renew a steadfast spirit within me.
Do not cast me from your presence
    or take your Holy Spirit from me.
Restore to me the joy of your salvation
    and grant me a willing spirit to sustain me.
Then I will teach transgressors your ways,
    and sinners will turn back to you.

—Psalm 51:10–13

O God, you are my God,
    earnestly I seek you;
my soul thirsts for you,
    my body longs for you,
in a dry and weary land
    where there is no water…
On my bed I remember you;
    I think of you through the watches of the night.
Because you are my help,
    I sing in the shadow of your wings.

—Psalm 63:1, 6–7

Teach us to number our days aright,
    that we may gain a heart of wisdom.

—Psalm 90:12

Praise the Lord, O my soul,
    and forget not all his benefits.

—Psalm 103:2

The Lord is with me; I will not be afraid.
    What can man do to me?

—Psalm 118:6

You will go out in joy
    and be led forth in peace;
the mountains and hills
    will burst into song before you,
and all the trees of the field
    will clap their hands.

—Isaiah 55:12

Surely I am with you always, to the very end of the age.
—Matthew 28:20

Whoever is thirsty, let him come; and whoever wishes, let him take the free gift of the water of life.
—Revelation 22:17

He tends his flock like a shepherd:
    He gathers the lambs in his arms
and carries them close to his heart;
    he gently leads those that have young.
—Isaiah 40:11

Endure hardship as discipline; God is treating you as sons... No discipline seems pleasant at the time, but painful. Later on, however, it produces a harvest of righteousness and peace for those who have been trained by it.
—Hebrews 12:7, 11

Consider it pure joy, my brothers, whenever you face trials of many kinds, because you know that the testing of your faith develops perseverance. Perseverance must finish its work so that you may be mature and complete, not lacking anything.
—James 1:2–4

He gives strength to the weary
　　and increases the power of the weak.
Even youths grow tired and weary,
　　and young men stumble and fall;
but those who hope in the Lord
　　will renew their strength.
They will soar on wings like eagles;
　　they will run and not grow weary,
　　they will walk and not be faint.

—Isaiah 40:29–31

It was good for me to be afflicted
　　so that I might learn your decrees.

—Psalm 119:71

Be still before the Lord and wait patiently for him...
　　For evil men will be cut off,
but those who hope in the Lord will inherit the land.

—Psalm 37:7, 9

The Lamb at the center of the throne will be their shepherd; he will lead them to springs of living water. And God will wipe away every tear from their eyes.

—Revelation 7:17

Appendix A

~

Resources to Use
in Doing Well

Some trust in chariots and some in horses,
but we trust in the name of the LORD *our God.*

PSALM 20:7

Organizations that Support People with Chronic Illness

One thing that those of us with chronic illness should realize right away is that we are not in this struggle alone. Many have walked this path before us and many are walking it now. A number of excellent organizations exist that can provide the information you need to do well. Some offer newsletters, some magazines, some online information, and some support groups. Explore these resources to arm yourself for the daily battles you will face.

The American Heart Association/American Stroke Association

7272 Greenville Avenue, Dallas, TX 75231
1-800 AHA-USA1 / 1-888-4-STROKE
www.americanheart.org

Information and research support for heart and stroke patients, including *Heart Insight* magazine and online heart encyclopedia.

American Lung Association

1301 Pennsylvania Ave., NW, Suite 800,
Washington, DC 20004
1-800-LUNG-USA
www.lungusa.org

Provides information and support for persons with asthma and other lung diseases and successfully lobbies for legal protections for clean air and breathing environments.

The Arthritis Foundation

P.O. Box 7669, Atlanta, GA 30357-0669
1-800-283-7800
www.arthritis.org

Excellent source of information, publishing books, booklets, and magazines, as well as participating in legislative efforts.

Lupus Alliance of America/Lupus Foundation of Western New York

3871 Harlem Road, Buffalo, NY 14215
1-866-415-8787
www.lupusalliance.org

Primarily a support organization that disperses information to its members through newsletters and local groups.

The National Fibromyalgia Association

2121 S. Towne Centre Place, Suite 300, Anaheim, CA 92806
1-714-921-0150
www.FMaware.org

A prime mover in bringing awareness and acceptance of the diagnosis of fibromyalgia and providing information to physicians and patients.

National Health Information Center (Nhic)

1-800-336-4797

A toll-free telephone referral service to organizations and resources that give specific information about many diseases.

Internet Resources

The Internet gives us unbelievable access to information. However, not all of the information is accurate. When you have received a diagnosis of a major illness, you will want to learn more about it, but you must be careful to search in places where the data has been checked for accuracy. I urge you not to spend time in chat rooms about illnesses, where participants often merely pool their ignorance and list symptoms. If you have hours to spend, use them at one of the sites that is well-respected in the medical community.

The Health On the Net Foundation (HON) provides a code of conduct for medical and health Web sites under which organizations can apply for accreditation. You would do well to evaluate the sites you mine for information based on HON criteria. In brief, the code insists that accredited sites be or have:

1. Authoritative—including the qualifications of the authors
2. Complementary—information should support rather than replace the doctor-patient relationship
3. Privacy—the site should respect the privacy and confidentiality of personal data submitted by the visitor
4. Attribution—the Web site should cite the sources and dates of published information
5. Justifiability—the site must back up claims related to benefits and performance
6. Transparency—the presentation should be accessible and the e-mail contact accurate
7. Financial disclosure—the site should identify its funding sources
8. Advertising policy—the site should clearly distinguish advertising from editorial content

(Source: Health On the Net Foundation, http://www.hon.ch/HONcode/Conduct.html)

Sites That You Might Find Helpful:

www.americanheart.org
Offers a monthly e-mail letter as well as well-organized information for heart and stroke patients.

www.cancer.gov
The Web site for the National Cancer Institute with links to research.

www.cancer.org
From the American Cancer Society, including links to support groups and research trials.

www.cdc.gov
From the Center for Disease Control and Prevention, providing timely information for the public concerning public health and communicable diseases.

www.clinicaltrials.gov
National listing of clinical trials of new treatments for various diseases.

www.diabetes.org
The American Diabetes Association gives news of research and practical information for diabetics.

www.familydoctor.org
Advice from the American Academy of Family Physicians about common questions they answer in their offices.

www.healthfinder.gov
Provides links to many sites containing reliable health care information from the US Department of Health and Human Services, in both English and Spanish.

www.healthywomen.org
Operated by the National Women's Health Resource Center, this site offers information on women's health issues, from dealing with the flu to questioning new ob-gyn treatments.

www.lungusa.org
Web site for the American Lung Association, offering information on all kinds of breathing issues, from asthma to air
quality.

www.mayoclinic.com
Excellent source of information on hundreds of medical topics.

http://www.medlineplus.gov
Large database from the National Library of Medicine cov-
ering most major illnesses, including definitions and basic
treatment options.

www.menopause.org
Good advice from the North American Menopause Society.

www.nih.gov
Online database of information about clinical trials being
held all over the United States.

www.patientinform.org
Offers links which describe the latest research of many medical organizations and gives free access to medical journal
articles.

www.quickenmedical.com
This software is not free, but it may pay for itself by aiding
you in the process of keeping track of what you have spent
and whether you have been reimbursed, as well as marking
purchases that are eligible for Flexible Spending Accounts.

www.simohealth.com
Software which is similar in design to the quickenmedical,
and which includes sections on dealing with insurance dis-
putes.

www.sleepfoundation.org
Sleep is often a problem for those with chronic illness, and
this site offers advice.

www.webmd.com
An information service which is for-profit rather than run by a non-profit organization and includes advertising as well as free information. Can include a daily newsletter which highlights top health stories.

Magazines and Newsletters

Arthritis Today
1330 West Peachtree St., NW, Suite 100, Atlanta, GA 30309
www.arthritis.org

Published six times a year, including an annual issue about medications and supplements useful in treating various forms of arthritis, this magazine sets the standard for self-help and research reviews.

Consumer Reports on Health
Box 5385, Harlan, IA 51593-0885
www.ConsumerReports.org/crh

Monthly digest of interesting articles about current health topics, from nutrition to surgeries. Well written and useful information.

Fibromyalgia Aware
2200 N. Glassell Street, Suite A, Orange, CA 92865
www.FMaware.org

Quarterly magazine providing research information and practical strategies for coping with fibromyalgia.

HEART INSIGHT Magazine
www.HeartInsight.com

Excellent resource highlighting research and heart healthy living, in English or Spanish.

Lunghealth
61 Broadway, New York, NY 10006-2701
www.lungusa.org

Publishers of *LUNG health*, a quarterly journal for those suffering from various diseases of the lung which offers practical suggestions as well as research news.

The Lupus Newslink
3871 Harlem Road, Buffalo, NY 14215
1-866-415-8787
www.lupusalliance.org

Bi-monthly newsletter includes information about the activities of chapter affiliates, practical advice, and research summaries.

The Mayo Clinic Health Letter
P.O. Box 9302, Big Sandy, TX 75755-9302
www.MayoClinic.com

Monthly newsletter that focuses on three or four topics and includes a question and answer section. Written by the well-respected Mayo Clinic.

Tufts University Health and Nutrition Letter
P.O. Box 5656, Norwalk, CT 06856-5656
www.healthletter.tufts.edu

Subtitled *Your Guide to Living Healthier Longer,* this monthly letter highlights recent research on diet and exercise, as well as spotlighting new drugs and supplements.

Books and Booklets

Bauer, Brent, M.D., ed. *The Mayo Clinic Book of Alternative Medicine.* New York: Time Inc., 2007.

An excellent blending of the finest in traditional and alternative medicine, with sections on herbs, minerals, mind-body medicine, energy and hands-on therapies, and other approaches to many common chronic conditions, including a section on finding qualified practitioners and working with your medical doctor to find alternatives when traditional medicine by itself is not optimal for your condition.

Beach, Shelly. *Precious Lord, Take My Hand.* Grand Rapids, MI: Discovery House Publishers, 2007.

A moving and helpful account of a couple's dedication to caring for their aging and ill parents by relying on God's guidance and grace.

Bhatt, Deepak, M.D., ed. *Coronary Artery Disease: Advances in Detection and Treatment.* Norwalk, CT: Cleveland Clinic, Health Special Reports, 2007.

An excellent compilation of information about CAD, from recent research to trends in treatment.

Cleveland Clinic and the editors of *Heart Advisor. Special Reports, including Coronary Artery Disease, 200, Advances in Detection and Treatment, Stroke: Advances in Treatment* and *Heart Failure: Advances in Prevention and Treatment.* Norwalk, CT: Health Special Reports, 2007.

The renowned Cleveland Clinic Heart Center provides overviews of the latest information on heart-related issues, including preventing future problems and accessing the latest in treatments. Updated yearly and written for the layperson to understand.

Donne, John. *Devotions upon Emergent Occasions.*

Written in 1630 and still a classic chronical of one believer's dealing with his impending death from both physical and religious perspectives. Donne's honesty and clarity compel the reader to share his journey.

Gruman, Jessie, Ph.D. *After Shock: What to Do When the Doctor Gives You—or Someone You Love—a Devastating Diagnosis,* Walker and Company, 2007.

A book for coping with the physical and emotional fall-out that occurs when you find you have a life-threatening illness written by a woman who has survived cancer and heart disease. Much practical advice.

Guarneri, Mimi, M.D. *The Heart Speaks: A Cardiologist Reveals the Secret Language of Healing.* New York: Touchstone Books, 2006.

A fascinating and informative book chronicling noted cardiologist Mimi Guarneri's growing appreciation of the non-medical factors in healing.

Hobbs, Robert E., M.D. *Heart Failure: Advances in Prevention and Treatment—2007 Report.* Norwalk, CT: Cleveland Clinic, Health Special Reports, 2007.

Offered by one of the premier cardiac teams in the nation, this booklet offers an overview of the disease with advances in treatment outlined clearly for the layperson.

Hoekstra, Elizabeth and Mary Bradford. *Chronic Kids, Constant Hope.* Crossway Books and Bible, 2000.

Two mothers' experiences in raising children with chronic illness, with strength-building results.

Larimore, Walt, M.D. with Traci Mullins. *God's Design for the Highly Healthy Person.* Grand Rapids, MI: Zondervan, 2003.

Endorsed by the Christian Medical Association, this book presents the answers to such questions as "What does it mean to be highly healthy?" and "What choices do I need to consider to create a more balanced lifestyle?" Drawing on a wealth of medical and practical knowledge as well as a strong spiritual base, Dr. Larimore has produced an excellent resource for encouraging health.

Also by Dr. Larimore and Donal O'Mathuna: *Alternative Medicine: The Christian Handbook*. Grand Rapids, MI: Zondervan, 2001.

A comprehensive guide to alternative treatments written from a distinctively Christian perspective which evaluates the claims and effectiveness of alternative therapies and remedies.

Lewis, C. S. *The Problem of Pain*. San Francisco: HarperCollins Publishers, 1940.

As only Lewis can, he clearly presents the arguments concerning the nature of God and the presence of pain in the world as we know it. Everyone should read this.

Mayo Clinic. *On* series. Rochester, MN: Mayo Clinic.

A set of books on various topics that presents the latest and best research clearly and understandably. Approachable and excellent.

Includes the following topics:
Alzheimer's Disease
Arthritis
Chronic Pain
Depression
Digestive Health
Healthy Aging
Healthy Weight
Heart Book
High Blood Pressure

Managing Diabetes
Mayo Clinic/Williams Sonoma Cookbook
Prostate Health
Self-Care
Vision and Eye Health.

Moffat, Marilyn and Steve Vickery. *The American Physical Therapy Association Book of Body Maintenance and Repair.* (New York: Owl Books, 1999).

An excellent resource for all who are trying to keep their bodies in working order, including sections on the proper working of all joints of the body and exercises to keep them functioning as well as possible.

Reisser, Paul, Dale Mabe, and Robert Velarde. *Examining Alternative Medicine: An Inside Look at the Benefits and Risks.* Downers Grove, IL: InterVarsity Press, 2001.

An excellent compendium of knowledge based on decades of practice and research by the authors. This book gives the reader a framework within which to evaluate alternative treatment options, including discussion of spiritual bases which may be at odds with biblical teaching.

Roizen, Michael and John LaPuma. *The RealAge Diet: Make Yourself Younger with What You Eat.* New York: Harper Collins, 2001.

Roizen, Michael and Mehmet Oz. *You: The Smart Patient: An Insider's Handbook for Getting the Best Treatment.* New York: Harper Collins, 2006.

Roizen, Michael and Mehmet Oz. *You on a Diet: Owner's Manual for Waist Management.* Harper Collins, New York, NY. 2006

These titles are accessible, humorous, and full of excellent information for all of us who "own" bodies.

Sim, Kay Tee and Bill Crowder. *Why Is Life So Unfair?* Grand Rapids, MI: Discovery House Publishers, 2007.

> One of the well-known Discovery Series Bible studies, this compilation of five Discovery Series booklets helps the reader come to grips with the presence of evil in the world from a biblical perspective.

Trent, John. *Strong Families in Stressful Times.* Harvest House, 2004.

> Trent once again gives families good lessons in building faith through times of trial.

Appendix B:

Becoming Real to Your Medical Team

OUR SECOND CESAREAN:
WHY WE FOUGHT TO HAVE MY HUSBAND THERE

(Condensed from Redbook Magazine, August 1979)

by Wendy Wallace

That baby will probably be born by lunch, and certainly before dinner. See you at the hospital." It was 9 a.m. when our obstetrician sent my husband Rick and me to the hospital to cope with labor pains together using the natural-childbirth techniques we had learned and await the birth of our first child.

At 4:30 the next morning the doctors told us that our baby was in distress, I would need surgery, and Rick must leave us. At 5:30 a.m. our nine-pound-five-ounce daughter, Carey, was delivered by cesarean section. The shock of being told I would need a surgical delivery left both of us feeling out of control. Having to be separated from Rick made everything more frightening for both of us. Rick sat outside the surgery room on the floor by himself, crying, because he thought my life was in jeopardy.

Finally the surgery was over, and we were reunited. Coming out of anesthesia, I was exhausted and in great pain, having been through twenty-four hours of labor with no food or sleep followed by two hours of abdominal surgery. But at least Rick and I were with each other again. Still, I made a mental vow not to have another child.

The final disappointment was that Carey's lungs were infected with strep, so she was in the Newborn Special Care Unit and was not allowed to be with me. Carey was the only reward I had for all this pain, and I couldn't even look at her or hold her.

During my hospital recovery I was exhausted, frustrated, and depressed. After nine months of eating spinach, taking my vitamins, and exercising daily, I thought my body was in shape to have the perfect Lamaze baby. Rick and I had learned how to breathe together, studied the stages of labor, and compared techniques with other parents. *Why had my body let me down?*

On top of that, I had been looking forward to being in control of my body again and instead found myself hooked up to an IV on one end and a catheter on the other. I could barely sit up by myself and walked only with extreme pain. My incision was infected with strep from the amniotic fluid, which had become contaminated during my long labor. The infection hung on, Carey and I were in the hospital for a month, and we began to doubt that I would be able to return to graduate school in the fall as we had planned. The difficult recovery reaffirmed my decision that Carey would be an only child. Rick accepted my decision.

Our daughter was a delightful person, and we both grew immeasurably from knowing her. We believed we were good parents, raising the kind of child we felt the world needed. And Carey enjoyed the company of other children so much that it became hard to think of her never having a sister or brother.

We began to talk about Carey's birth and rethink the possibilities. Her large size had necessitated a cesarean section, and if we had another baby, he or she also would probably have to be delivered surgically. But neither of us could understand why this should mean we had to be separated while our child was born. We decided to have another child and do everything possible to be together at the birth.

As soon as I got pregnant we visited Henry Magendantz, the obstetrician who had delivered Carey. He was very supportive of our plan. Other hospitals across the country were allowing fathers at cesarean deliveries, and we all thought that Yale-New Haven Hospital, connected to a prestigious university, would want to be a leader in this. He approached the director of obstetrics and was told that although the hospital received four or five requests such as ours weekly, the plan was impossible. Thus began our nine-month fight with the university hospital.

First we wrote a letter to the head of the department of obstetrics to open communications. Our official request was that we be a test case. We sent the department head the guidelines prepared by Boston Hospital for Women, a pioneer in this area.

Almost seventeen percent of births today are cesareans, and most couples, like us, never anticipate the necessity for the surgery. Non-planned cesareans are often accompanied by feelings of anger, guilt, and inadequacy in both the mother and father. The mothers feel that if they had been better prepared they somehow could have avoided this painful, difficult, nonfamily birth. Fathers feel helpless to alleviate their wives' suffering.

Research shows that for many of these couples a primary source of pain is the fact that just when they need each other the most, the father is asked to leave. Their separation sets the stage for the lack of communication that follows.

We contacted C/SEC, a Boston-based organization providing information and support for those who undergo or anticipate a cesarean. Just as useful as their information was the attitude of the C/SEC staff, who regard a cesarean as a birth, not an operation. With this in mind, our emotional preparation for my delivery became much more positive.

From the thoughtful, caring women at C/SEC, all of whom had had a cesarean at some time, we learned that Boston Hospital for Women had done over a thousand cesareans with the father present and that only a few fathers had fainted—one of our hospital's stated objections. Other than this, they found no ill effects and many benefits, including mothers using less anesthesia during the birth and fewer painkillers during recovery and babies growing faster than those whose mothers had undergone the operation alone.

We knew from personal experience that having the father present was *emotionally* superior, but this information indicated that it was *medically* superior, and we hoped it would convince the medical staff at Yale-New Haven. We contacted the chiefs of obstetrics and anesthesiology at Boston Hospital and asked them to write to our hospital and describe the results of their policy, which they did gladly. We also asked permission to speak to the obstetrics faculty at the hospital.

Ultimately the decision was put to a vote of the senior faculty—mostly older men who had not been exposed to our barrage of information and to whom we had not been allowed to speak. Through our many new friends in the hospital system we learned that our request had been denied, but that more faculty had voted for it than the chairman had expected.

Though we were not even officially informed of the meeting, we knew what had happened and began to feel there was no hope. Time was running out. Perhaps we should consider going to another hospital, even though it would mean leaving our own obstetrician. After much hard thinking we decided that Rick's presence was so important to us that we would rather have someone else delivery our baby at an accommodating hospital than miss Rick's being there. Dr. Magendantz contacted a colleague who was affiliated with a hospital fifty miles away where we would be allowed to have a family birth. We made an appointment to see the new doctor four days before the baby was due.

In a last attempt, we decided to inform the university president's office about our request and the fact that we had not received any official response. We had much support in the community by this time, and we hoped the university might use its influence to persuade the obstetrics department.

Several days later Rick made a final phone call to the head of obstetrics to restate our case. The news he received was stunning: the faculty members had changed their minds! We didn't believe it until we received the permission in writing.

On our due date, instead of meeting a new doctor at a new hospital, we checked into Yale-New Haven hospital. I was prepped and Rick got dressed in his funny-looking surgical gown and slippers. I was nervous, but not afraid as I had been at Carey's birth. I knew that if there were any unexpected problems during surgery, Rick would be there as my protector and advocate to watch out for me, to help make the kind of decisions I would have made.

At 10:40 a.m. our nine-pound-seven-ounce son, Mark, was born. I could not see him because of the sterile drape over my abdomen, but I could see Rick's face burst into a smile. As the baby was lifted up, he yelled, "It's a boy!" We both laughed and cried.

Mark was taken to the pediatrics table, examined, cleaned a little, wrapped up, and placed in Rick's arms. Our baby screamed lustily, and we sang him lullabies. The anesthesiologist, who had been a tremendous support throughout the process, unstrapped one of my arms, and I touched my son, feeling his newborn softness and marveling that only minutes before he had been a part of my body. I was absolutely elated.

The joy we felt filled the entire room. We smiled and kissed and said how much he looked like various relatives. We debated whether he was a baritone or a tenor. But most important, we welcomed him into the love we felt for each other and began a loving relationship that will stay with him for life.

I healed very quickly with no infection. Although I had pain, C/SEC had taught me how to cope with it, and I knew that it would end soon. Since we both were in good shape Mark was with me continuously, bolstering my spirits with every smile and gurgle. This time I was not angry with my body, and except for a brief bout with post-partum blues, I had no depression at all.

After that experience I was surer than ever that couples should be able to have their babies together. Such a significant moment in their lives cannot be fully shared in words after it has occurred. The feelings that come during the birth must be experienced. Further, the assurance of love from both parents that the child receives, and the reassurance of love that the parents give to each other, are two of the intangible and invaluable rewards of a family birth.

Now Rick and I teach couples who anticipate possible cesarean sections. We speak of our experiences as well as those of the many cesarean couples we have come to know. Our groups include mothers with high blood pressure, diabetes, tumors or cysts, plus those who expect twins, babies in the breech position, or babies who are very large compared to the size of the mother's pelvis. Research has shown that these mothers experience less depression, anger, and difficulty accepting the cesarean birth if they know what to expect. But that should not be surprising, since we all handle adversity better if we are prepared for it.

The husbands and wives in class remind me of us in many ways: anxious, suspicious, and afraid of the unknown. But because of our fight and the efforts of many other parents and professionals who believe in family birth, they now have the option of facing that unknown together. It is sometimes difficult to answer their questions, especially when they hit upon something that was physically or emotionally painful to us. But the couples are always encouraged when they hear the description of Rick as he watched Mark being born. Once again I see the smile that seems to come from his entire being, and once again I laugh and cry at the same time.

~

For information from C/SEC and help in locating any of 175 affiliated groups, write C/SEC, 66 Christopher Road, Waltham, Massachusetts 02154.

Note to the Reader

~

The publisher invites you to share your response to the message of this book by writing Discovery House Publishers, P.O. Box 3566, Grand Rapids, MI 49501, U.S.A. For information about other Discovery House books, music, videos, or DVDs, contact us at the same address or call 1-800-653-8333. Find us on the Internet at http://www.dhp.org/ or send an e-mail to books@dhp.org.